Essential endocrinology

Julius Lee
Late Professor of Endocrine Physiology, Charing Cross Hospital Medical School

John Laycock
Lecturer, Department of Physiology, Charing Cross Hospital Medical School

1978

OXFORD UNIVERSITY PRESS

Oxford   New York   Toronto

Oxford University Press, Walton Street,
Oxford ox2 6DP

Oxford London Glasgow
New York Toronto Melbourne Wellington
Ibadan Nairobi Dar es Salaam Lusaka Cape Town
Kuala Lumpur Singapore Jakarta Hong Kong Tokyo
Delhi Bombay Calcutta Madras Karachi

British Library Cataloguing in Publication Data
Lee, Julius
    Essential endocrinology. (Oxford medical publications.)
    1. Endocrinology
    I. Title   II. Series   III. Laycock, John F.
    616.4   RC648   78-40066
ISBN 0-19-261123-2

Printed in Great Britain by Cox & Wyman Ltd,
London, Fakenham and Reading

Preface

Textbooks of endocrinology are usually written to accommodate the requirements of clinical students. This book is an attempt to provide sufficient information for medical students not only in their clinical but also in their preclinical years.

While it is appreciated that physiological and clinical aspects of endocrinology are closely related, they are considered separately when possible. This approach allows for the concise presentation of information and leaves integration to the student. It is our hope that this book will be used as a basis upon which a true understanding of the subject can be achieved.

Chapter 11, entitled 'common endocrine emergencies', has been written primarily for use on the wards and may be particularly helpful at times when advice from senior colleagues is not readily available. The final chapter, on tests of endocrine function, is presented in a form which is intended to give easy reference to the appropriate tests, and is illustrated by examples which we hope will allow for an appreciation of the importance of their correct interpretation.

Students, past and present, have maintained our interest in endocrinology by their persistent questioning. This has encouraged us to extend our knowledge and to try to stay 'one step ahead'; in return, we dedicate this book to them.

It is a pleasure to record our thanks to those past and present members of the Endocrine Unit at Charing Cross Hospital who have contributed towards the various chapters: in particular, Dr. P. Dorrington Ward (Chapter 4); Mr. M. Pawson, Dr. Janet Lambley (née Booth), and Dr. T. Greenwood (Chapter 5); Dr. K. Waters (Chapters 6 and 7); Dr. A. L. Wyman (Chapter 8); Professor J. Daly and Mr. R. W. Hoile for material on ectopic secretion and the Zollinger–Ellison syndrome respectively (Chapter 9); Dr. A. Khaleeli (Chapter 11); and Dr. J. Alaghband-Zadeh (Chapter 12).

Clinical colleagues have read many of the chapters and attempted to correct errors and point out omissions. Among these are Professor Reginald Hall, who read and commented on several chapters, Dr. Jean Ginsberg (Royal Free Hospital), and Dr. Jean Ross, who read and commented on the draft of Chapter 5. Any remaining errors and omissions are entirely our own responsibility.

The clinical photographs form part of the endocrine unit collection and are presented with the consent of Professor Lee's consultant colleagues. We should like to express our gratitude to the patients for their kind permission to use the photographs and to the Department of Medical Illustration for the reproductions.

Finally our thanks are extended to secretaries Miss Amanda Watkins, Mrs. Hilary Dance, and Miss Alison Castledine, all of whom have patiently typed the various stages of the manuscript.

September 1977   J.L., J.F.L.

Professor Lee died without having the satisfaction of seeing this book in print. *Essential endocrinology* is a testimony to his dedicated work in the two fields of his special choosing, the science of endocrinology and the art of teaching.

November 1977   J.F.L.

Contents

1 Introduction

Plan of this book

The sequence of this book has been deliberately selected. The hypothalamus is considered first (in Chapter 2) because this is an important example of a nervous tissue which secretes hormones; furthermore this structure is essential for the normal activity of the hypophysis (pituitary gland) which is discussed in the same chapter. It may appear strange that the chapter on adrenal medulla is interposed between this chapter and those three chapters which consider the endocrine glands which are dependent upon the adenohypophysis (anterior pituitary). By adopting this particular order however, we enable the reader to consider first those endocrine glands which are mainly controlled by the nervous system and subsequently those endocrine glands which are influenced by the adenohypophysis. The parathyroids and the islets of Langerhans have to be discussed separately since their hormones are controlled mainly by the concentrations of those particular chemical substances which they themselves regulate.

We have included a variety of aspects in Chapter 9 ('miscellaneous subjects'), such as the concept of 'amine precursor uptake decarboxylation' cells (APUD cells), ectopic secretion, multiple endocrine adenomatosis, tumours of the (δ) islet cells, and consideration of two important substances: 5 hydroxytryptamine (including carcinoid) and prostaglandins, which are not easily classified but which are of importance to the clinical student. Chapter 10 has been devoted to a brief consideration of some common intracellular mechanisms through which many hormones are now believed to act. Chapter 11 is intended principally for the newly qualified graduate. The final Chapter (12) provides not only immediate reference to the appropriate tests of endocrine function, but also to the essential technical problems involved in some of these measurements, enabling the reader to assess their relative importance.

Certain tissues which can be considered to have an endocrine function have been excluded. While it is difficult to defend the exclusion of the upper part of the alimentary canal, this together with the spleen, the kidney, the thymus and the pineal gland have been omitted in accordance with many other textbooks. It is of interest to note that the thymus has now become a prized possession of the immunologist.

Each chapter concerned with a particular endocrine gland (Chapters 2–8 inclusive) has been written in two parts: the basic physiology of the gland is considered first (including a brief section on its general anatomy, histology, and development), followed by consideration of the clinical disorders associated with that gland. Naturally there is some interchange between the physiological and clinical components where necessary allowing both the preclinical and clinical student to appreciate the importance of physiology in medicine.

History

In 1905 Starling first applied the word 'hormone' to secretin, a chemical secreted into the blood-stream which stimulated the flow of pancreatic fluid. Subsequently a hormone was defined as 'any substance normally produced in the cells of some part of the body and carried by the blood-stream to distant parts which it affects for the good of the body as a whole'. Thus an endocrine gland was defined as a normal tissue which is ductless, and which secretes chemical messengers—the hormones—directly into the blood. Some tissues which secrete hormones, for instance the alimentary canal, are frequently omitted from textbooks of endocrinology, possibly because of their lack of interest to the clinical endocrinologist. This has resulted in confusion about the definition of an endocrine gland.

The belief that endocrine glands are secretors of chemical messengers which enter the blood-stream to affect the activity of other tissues provoked adverse criticism until the beginning of the twentieth century. However, evidence for this concept was rapidly accumulated from the scientific field aided and indeed stimulated by clinical observations, some of which had been made in the nineteenth century.

The appreciation of such a system, then, stimulated various disciplines. To the evolutionist the endocrine system could be accepted as a natural auxillary to the central nervous system (CNS). As the complexity of the organism developed (to include a cardiovascular system), it became essential that the response to a stimulus could be prolonged. In these circumstances the CNS, which in general evokes a rapid response, would be inefficient, whereas chemical messengers in the blood-stream could prolong a response, enabling better adaptation to changes in the external environment. To the biologist the endocrine system represents a mechanism for controlling growth, maturation, metabolism, and reproduction in an organism. To the clinical endocrinologist a certain pattern of symptoms and signs elicited on examination could now be shown to be the result of a disorder of a particular endocrine gland. Endocrinology should encompass all these aspects; furthermore the endocrinologist should try to extend his knowledge to include, for example, the biochemistry of the intracellular actions of hormones.

In the early days of neurophysiology the function of the nervous system was regarded simply as conveying and modifying action potentials. In the invertebrates (e.g. insects) many hormones are released from 'neurohaemal' organs, which anatomically consist of nerve fibres in close contact with blood, enabling the nerve endings to release chemical substances which may then pervade the whole insect. It was then realized that vertebrate nerve cells similarly release chemical substances and if these cells are in close association with a capillary these substances can also be released directly into the blood-stream to act as hormones (neurosecretion). Neurosecretions which are not released into the blood-stream, but act locally, are called neurotransmitters.

Control of hormonal secretion

1. Feedback mechanisms

Some basic knowledge of feedback mechanisms is required in order to understand individual control systems in endocrinology, and they are therefore briefly considered here. This section may appear complex, but an early discussion on the importance of feedback mechanisms will prove useful to the reader who should, whenever necessary, refer back to this chapter.

The basic function of a hormone is to regulate the metabolic activity of its target cells in a specific direction. To maintain this function it is essential that the endocrine gland receives constant rapid information (feedback) on the state of those systems regulated. A simple feedback as described may be insufficient and usually an endocrine gland continually receives signals from a variety of different sources and the rate of hormonal secretion from the gland is therefore determined by the integration of these different afferent signals.

(a) Direct negative feedback

Probably the most simple feedback to an endocrine gland is the direct negative feedback system which relates the rate of release of the hormone to the blood concentration of that chemical substance which it controls (or to a chemical product of the metabolic process which it regulates). An example of this type of feedback mechanism is the relationship between the hormone insulin and the variable which it controls, the blood glucose concentration. Insulin acts upon its target cells ultimately to decrease blood glucose levels; a change in these levels in turn alters the rate of secretion of insulin. Thus a rise in blood glucose levels increases the rate of secretion of the hormone which then acts on its target to restore the blood glucose to normal levels (simple direct negative feedback mechanism).

Some hormones from the adenohypophysis (anterior pituitary) act primarily to regulate the secretions of other endocrine glands. For example hormone X' from the adenohypophysis acts upon an endocrine gland to stimulate the release of hormone X. This hormone can then influence its own release by direct negative feedback on the secretion of hormone X' from the adenohypophysis (see Fig. 1.1). An increase in the secretion of X' results in an increased release of X. Hormone X then acts on the adenohypophysis to inhibit the release of X' which, in turn, results in a decreased secretion of X. The blood level of X is thus regulated within narrow limits.

(b) Indirect negative feedback

This term is used when the central nervous system, in particular the hypothalamus, is indirectly involved in the regulation of hormone secretion from an endocrine gland by controlling the release of the appropriate adenohypophysial hormones. In such a system, hormone X from the target endocrine gland can have a direct negative feedback on the release of the adenohypophysial hormone X' (see previous section) and an indirect negative feedback on the release of the hypothalamic hormone X'' (see Fig. 1.2).

This indirect involvement of the hypothalamus is particularly important in the control of thyroidal, adrenocortical, and gonadal secretions (see relevant chapters).

Fig.1.1
Diagram illustrating the direct
negative (−ve) feedback which
can exist between the target
endocrine gland hormone X
and the release of the
adenohypophysial hormone
X′.

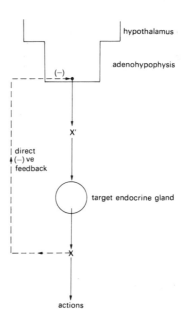

Fig.1.2
Diagram illustrating the direct
negative (−ve) feedback loop
which can exist between
hormone X from the target
endocrine gland and the
release of the
adenohypophysial hormone
X′, and the indirect negative
(−ve) feedback between X and
the hypothalamic hormone
X′′.

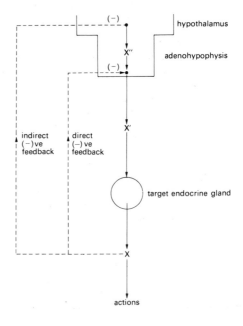

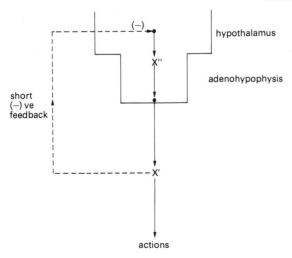

Fig.1.3 Diagram illustrating the short negative (−ve) feedback which can exist between the adenohypophysial hormone X′ and the release of the hypothalamic hormone X″.

(c) Short feedback

As mentioned previously, the hypothalamus controls the release of adenohypophysial hormones by secreting releasing (or release-inhibiting) substances. Some of the adenohypophysial hormones are believed to have a feedback effect on the release of the hypothalamic hormones and this type of regulating system is called a short feedback loop (see Fig. 1.3).

(d) Positive feedback

In addition to the various negative feedback mechanisms discussed, positive feedback systems exist in which the change elicited by the action of the hormone alters the rate of release of that hormone (or some other hormone) so that its effect is further enhanced. This type of feedback could rapidly become uncontrollable if there were no other control mechanisms involved in the system. One example of such a positive feedback mechanism is the release of oestrogens (the generic name for a group of female sex hormones) from the ovarian follicle, controlled by the adenohypophysial hormone follicle-stimulating hormone (FSH). At a particular plasma concentration oestrogen stimulates the release of more FSH and luteinizing hormone (LH) from the adenohypophysis, so that a positive feedback between oestrogens and FSH occurs which would be unstable if no other factors were involved (see Fig. 1.4). This positive feedback mechanism is also probably mediated partly through the hypothalamus (see Chapter 5).

2. The influence of the CNS

Some endocrine glands are controlled primarily by the nervous system: these are the neurohypophysis and the adrenal medulla. The adrenal medulla is an endocrine gland which is directly controlled by nerve impulses propagated

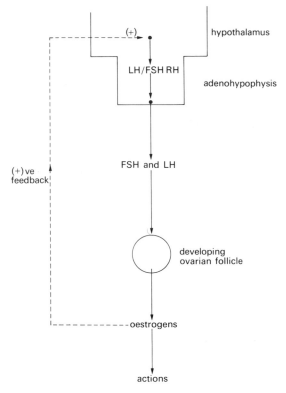

Fig.1.4   Diagram illustrating the positive feedback (+ve) which can exist between the plasma oestrogen concentration (at low levels) and the release of the adenohypophysial hormones FSH and LH.

along sympathetic preganglionic fibres originating in the hypothalamic region, with the ultimate mediation of a neurotransmitter (in this case acetylcholine) at the nerve terminals. Feedback in this čase is integrated with the general autonomic reflexes which originate in the hypothalamus. In this system, an increase in sympathetic activity results in an excitation of the cells of the adrenal medulla which then release adrenalin.

One mechanism controlling the release of the neurohypophysial hormone vasopressin involves changes in the frequency of nervous impulses along specific nerve pathways from blood volume receptors. This feedback mechanism involves a neurotransmitter acting on the cell bodies of those neurones originating mainly in the supra-optic nucleus of the hypothalamus (see Chapter 2) which synthesize, store, and release vasopressin (Fig. 1.5). When the volume receptors are stimulated (by volume expansion for instance) the tonic inhibition exerted by this feedback system is increased, and therefore vasopressin secretion is decreased.

The importance of the relationship between the nervous system and endo-

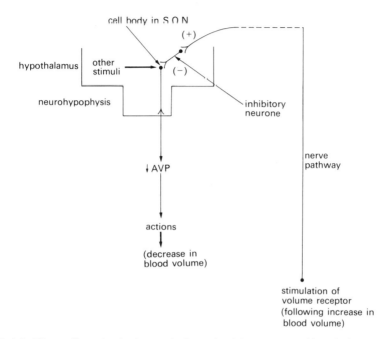

Fig.1.5 Diagram illustrating the decreased release of arginine-vasopressin (↓AVP) which results from increased stimulation of volume receptors following blood volume expansion (see text). S.O.N. = Supra-optic nucleus.

crine system is also emphasized through the various feedback control mechanisms which involve the hypothalamus. Since the hypothalamic nuclei also receive signals from other ('higher') centres in the brain, one special feature of the regulation of hypophysial hormone release is the ability of the brain to 'over-ride', or to finely adjust, all other control mechanisms. This type of control by the 'higher' centres of the brain is sometimes called 'an open-loop control system'.

Summary

The control of an endocrine gland's secretion is often complex and can involve not only nervous control loops but also chemical substances in the blood; these may be the actual concentrations of the hormones themselves. The close integration between nervous and endocrine systems is essential for the maintenance of a constant internal environment in the face of continually changing external conditions.

2 The hypothalamo-hypophysial system

PHYSIOLOGY

The hypothalamus and neurosecretions

The fundamental importance of the hypothalamus within the endocrine system was only appreciated following a series of experiments in the 1950s. This region of the brain is now considered as an endocrine gland in addition to its previously accepted functions, such as the regulation of autonomic nervous reflexes and temperature control.

Anatomy

The hypothalamus consists of nervous tissue below the thalamus. It virtually surrounds part of the third ventricle, with efferent and afferent fibres connecting it to the rest of the central nervous system. There are numerous groups of nerve cells (nuclei), but it is not yet possible to designate a specific function to the majority of these nuclei.

The hypothalamus is supplied with blood from the circle of Willis and, although most of the venous blood drains into the vein of Galen, a proportion flows through the capillary plexus in the median eminence to enter a sinusoidal network in the adenohypophysis (the anterior pituitary gland). The latter is an example of a venous portal system and is called the hypothalamo-hypophysial portal system (see Fig. 2.1).

The neurosecretions

Synthesis, storage, and release

The description now given is restricted to that part of the hypothalamus whose nerve cells have axons extending to the median eminence and the hypophysis

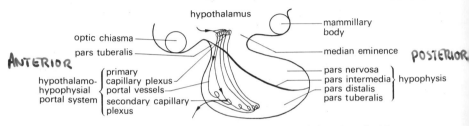

Fig.2.1   Diagram illustrating a cross-section of the hypothalamo-hypophysial system.

NEURAL HYPOPHYSIS. - Posterior
Median eminence
Infundibulum
Neural Lobe (pars nervosa)

ADENOHYPOPHYSIS - Anterior
Pars distalis
Pars intermedia
Pars tuberalis

(pituitary gland). It is now accepted that synthesis and storage of chemical substances takes place within specific hypothalamic nerve cells; furthermore the release of these chemicals occurs from nerve terminals in close association with blood-vessels. As these substances originate from nerve cells the term neurosecretion is employed, and these neurosecretions satisfy the criteria for classification as hormones. However, we shall apply the term 'hormone' only if the chemical structure is known, otherwise reference is made to hypothalamic factors. This arbitrary classification has found universal acceptance.

Of the various hypothalamic nuclei, most have all their nerve endings in the region of the median eminence, but two have the majority of their axons terminating in the posterior pituitary gland with relatively few fibres ending in the median eminence and pituitary stalk. This hypothalamic/posterior pituitary system is called the neurohypophysis, and its two neurosecretions are octapeptide hormones (see page 16).

The neurosecretions in the median eminence are released into the portal system to the adenohypophysis and so far three have been identified as small polypeptides. Little is known about the actual processes involved in the synthesis of many of these substances, although it is probable that this occurs in the cell bodies. Similarly, the storage of these substances may occur in the respective nerve terminals. It is not yet known whether they are stored as a bound complex, perhaps involving a larger protein molecule, or whether storage is in the free (unbound) form, in vesicles.

Each median eminence neurosecretion acts on particular adenohypophysial cells to influence the release of a specific adenohypophysial hormone. Only three of these neurosecretions have so far been identified: these are (1) thyrotrophin releasing hormone (TRH) which stimulates the release of thyrotrophin (thyroid stimulating hormone, TSH); (2) luteinizing hormone-releasing hormone (LHRH) which (see later) also appears to influence FSH release, and (3) somatostatin which is somatotrophin-inhibiting hormone.

The remaining adenohypophysial hormones are also influenced by releasing factors, and in some instances also by inhibiting factors. Corticotrophin (or adrenocorticotrophic hormone, ACTH) and melanocyte-stimulating hormone (MSH) are under the control of their respective releasing factors, while somatotrophin (growth hormone, GH) and prolactin appear to be controlled by both releasing and release-inhibiting factors, the latter being the dominating influence on prolactin release. With reference to follicle-stimulating hormone (FSH) there is some uncertainty as to whether control is by a specific releasing factor or whether luteinizing hormone-releasing hormone (LHRH) also controls its release, and reference is often made to FSH/LHRH. The release of any one of the releasing (or release-inhibiting) -hormones or factors from its particular hypothalamic nucleus is probably controlled in part by nervous impulses from other parts of the central nervous system. This would account for the important influence of external stimuli such as environmental changes, emotion, and stress on the release of certain adenohypophysial hormones. In addition hypothalamic endocrine activity is controlled by hormone feedback mechanisms (see Chapter 1) and to some degree influenced by the concentration of particular chemical substances in the blood.

The adenohypophysis and adenohypophysial hormones

The general physiological functions of the adenohypophysial hormones are briefly considered in this section. Greater detail may be given in other chapters which discuss those endocrine glands whose secretory activities are controlled by adenohypophysial hormones (i.e. thyroid, adrenal cortex, and gonads) together with greater detail concerning feedback, and other, control mechanisms. A general discussion on feedback control mechanisms was given in the Introduction (Chapter 1) and should be referred to when necessary.

Anatomy, histology, and development

The hypophysis (pituitary gland) lies in the sella turcica at the base of the brain. The adenohypophysis consists of the anterior part of the gland and comprises the pars distalis and the pars tuberalis. It develops from Rathke's pouch, an upgrowth of ectodermal cells from the roof of the primitive pharynx.

In man, the pars distalis receives most of its blood-supply from the anterior hypophysial artery in the hypothalamus. Arterial blood in a network of capillary loops (primary plexus) in the ventral hypothalamus drains into sinusoids which descend through the pituitary stalk to form a second capillary network (secondary plexus) in the pars distalis. This blood-system, which involves primary and secondary capillary plexuses connected by sinusoids, is called the hypothalamo-hypophysial portal system (see Fig. 2.1). The pars intermedia (intermediate lobe) is almost non-existent in man and is relatively avascular. The pars distalis is innervated with sympathetic and parasympathetic nerve fibres, but nervous connections with the hypothalamus are very scant.

Histologically three types of cell can be differentiated using standard staining techniques: acidophils, (or eosinophils), basophils, and chromophobes. Nearly 40 per cent of the cells are granular acidophils and some 10 per cent are granular basophils. The remaining 50 per cent are agranular chromophobes which in the past have been considered to be precursor cells of the acidophils and basophils. This classification of adenohypophysial cells is now generally considered to be too simple since it does not account for the specific synthesis and release of at least six different hormones. Nor does it adequately explain how some chromophobe-cell tumours may secrete large amounts of adenohypophysial hormones.

The seven principal hormones from the adenohypophysis can be considered in two groups: those which have their primary effect on other tissues directly, and those whose primary effect is to stimulate other endocrine glands to secrete their hormones (see Table 2.1).

The adenohypophysial hormones

1. Somatotrophin

Somatotrophin is a small protein which, in man, consists of 191 amino acids. Its molecular weight is approximately 27 000 and it has two disulphide bridges. It is synthesized in acidophilic cells and stored in intracellular granules. It is released into the blood by exocytosis. In adults the rate of secretion is variable

Table 2.1   The adenohypophysial hormones

Hormones acting primarily on target tissues:
1. somatotrophin (growth hormone, GH)
2. prolactin
3. melanocyte-stimulating hormone (MSH)

Hormones acting primarily on target endocrine glands (trophic hormones):
1. thyrotrophin (thyroid-stimulating hormone, TSH)
2. corticotrophin (adrenocorticotrophic hormone, ACTH)
3. gonadotrophins
    i. luteinizing hormone (LH); also called interstitial-cell stimulating hormone, ICSH, in males
    ii. follicle-stimulating hormone (FSH)

---

during each 24 hours with a normal daily output around 1·4 mg. In the circulation, two discrete components have been identified; the smaller component is possibly a breakdown product.

Actions

The most noticeable effect of somatotrophin is the promotion of growth which it induces in many soft tissues, in cartilage and bone. This action results from the stimulation of protein synthesis which is partly induced by an enhancement of amino acid transport through cell membranes. The effects on linear growth are now believed to be mediated by a hormone which is synthesized in the liver and kidneys under the influence of somatotrophin. This mediator is a peptide (mol. wt approximately 4000) and is called somatomedin.

The increase in the growth of soft and skeletal tissues induced by somatotrophin is accompanied by changes in electrolyte metabolism. The increase in protein synthesis results in a positive nitrogen and phosphorus balance, while blood urea levels fall. The intestinal absorption of calcium is increased and the urinary excretion of sodium and potassium fall probably resulting from the increased uptake of these ions by the growing tissues. Somatotrophin stimulates the uptake of non-esterified fatty acids (NEFA) by muscle and causes a significant but delayed increase in the mobilization of NEFA from adipose tissue. The hormone influences lipolysis through the mediation of cAMP. Somatotrophin also stimulates hepatic glycogenolysis and antagonizes the effect of insulin (see Chapter 8) on glucose uptake by peripheral cells, so that the blood glucose concentration can increase. The roles of somatotrophin and insulin are complementary in inducing growth since they both have protein anabolic effects and stimulate the transport of amino acids into peripheral cells, while their respective effects on the blood-glucose level will tend to oppose each other. If excess somatotrophin is released due to an acidophil-adenoma, it may cause hyperglycaemia which can become permanent (diabetes mellitus).

The control of release

The release of somatotrophin from the adenohypophysis is primarily under the control of two hypothalamic factors released into the portal blood-system from

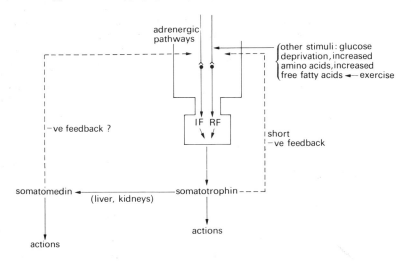

Fig.2.2 Diagram illustrating the principal control mechanisms involved in the release of somatotrophin (growth hormone) from the adenohypophysis. A possible negative feedback by somatomedin is indicated.

nerve terminals in the median eminence. One factor stimulates the release of somatotrophin while the other, less important, factor called somatostatin inhibits its release. Somatostatin has been found not only in the hypothalamus but also in the delta (δ) cells of the pancreatic islets of Langerhans (see Chapter 8). Control over the release of the two hypothalamic factors appears to be primarily from the higher centres of the brain, although important feedback mechanisms do exist. Various stimuli such as emotional, febrile, and surgical stresses probably affect their release directly from the higher centres through the activation of an adrenergic system. Other factors such as levels of energy substrate in the blood, in particular hypoglycaemia, increased amino acid levels (in particular arginine) and fatty acids all appear to stimulate somatotrophin release, possibly through the adrenergic system. In addition, the blood level of circulating somatotrophin is thought to exert an influence on the release of the hypothalamic factors through a short feedback loop, and somatomedin may also have a negative feedback at hypothalamic and/or adenohypophysial levels (Fig. 2.2).

2. Prolactin

Prolactin is a protein whose chemical structure is similar to that of somatotrophin. It has 170 amino acids and its molecular weight is approximately 25 000. It is synthesized and stored in acidophil cells. The only established function for prolactin is the initiation and maintenance of lactation in females, and even for this one action to be effective requires the presence of various other hormones such as oestrogens, corticosteroids, and insulin. General metabolic functions similar to those of somatotrophin have also been observed, but the importance of prolactin for these effects is unclear. As yet no known function for prolactin has been established in males.

Prolactin release is under the control of the hypothalamus which receives afferent impulses initiated from sensory receptors on the breasts and especially round the nipples in females. A hypothalamic inhibitory factor appears to be more dominant than the releasing factor. Unexpectedly thyrotrophin-releasing hormone also appears to be able to stimulate the release of prolactin, although the physiological significance of this action remains unclear.

3. Melanocyte-stimulating hormone

The hypophysis contains two melanocyte-stimulating hormones (α and βMSH). The βMSH is a polypeptide of 22 amino acids whose structure is similar to part of the corticotrophin molecule. It appears to be released in parallel with corticotrophin, and may account for the heavy pigmentation which is often a symptom of excessive corticotrophin release. The only known function in man is to increase pigmentation of the skin by increasing melanin synthesis in the melanocytes. The melanin appears to be able to move out of these cells in humans, and is then dispersed in the surrounding dermal cells. Other effects have been claimed (e.g. on the nervous system) but their physiological significance is unknown. Its release is believed to be controlled by the same hypothalamic releasing factor which stimulates corticotrophin release (CRF).

4. Thyrotrophin

Thyrotrophin is a glycoprotein hormone which is synthesized and stored in particular basophilic cells of the adenohypophysis. Its primary action is to stimulate the thyroid gland to secrete two of its own hormones, tri-iodothyronine (T_3) and thyroxine (T_4) into the blood-stream. This action of thyrotrophin on the thyroid gland is the result of several different effects on the intracellular mechanisms involved in the synthesis and release of the thyroidal metabolic hormones. These effects are:

a. stimulation of the iodide pump in the cell membrane which transports iodide from the blood into the cells against an electrochemical gradient;

b. stimulation of the synthesis of the thyroidal storage protein thyroglobulin;

c. stimulation of T_3 and T_4 synthesis;

d. stimulation of the release of T_3 and T_4 from the thyroglobulin complexes.

In addition the follicular cells increase in size and number resulting in an enlarged thyroid gland (goitre). Thyrotrophin may also have extrathyroidal effects such as the lipolysis induced in isolated tissues but the physiological importance of such actions is unclear.

5. Corticotrophin

This hormone is a polypeptide of 39 amino acids which is synthesized and stored in particular basophilic cells of the adenohypophysis. Its primary function is to stimulate the two innermost zones of the cortex of the adrenal gland, the zonae fasciculata and reticularis, which secrete the glucocorticoid hormones (primarily cortisol in man) and small quantities of sex hormones (androgens and oestrogens). It is also believed to sensitize the outermost zone of the adrenal cortex, the zona glomerulosa, to other stimuli which induce the release of the mineralocorticoid hormone aldosterone (see Chapter 4).

Its extra-adrenal effects are observed mainly when it is present in excess, resulting from a basophil adenoma for instance (Cushing's disease). These effects include some mobilization of fats following increased lipolysis, the stimulation of glucose and amino acid uptake by skeletal muscle, and stimulation of the release of insulin from the pancreatic islet cells and somatotrophin from the adenohypophysis. In addition, a markedly increased pigmentation is often observed, and this effect may be due to part of the corticotrophin molecule which is in part identical to melanocyte-stimulating hormone, MSH. However, as mentioned earlier, this effect may be due to an increased release of MSH itself.

6. Luteinizing hormone (LH)

This gonadotrophic hormone is also a glycoprotein molecule synthesized and stored in certain basophilic cells of the adenohypophysis. In females it acts primarily to precipitate ovulation by acting synergistically with FSH, and then maintains the secretory functions of the corpus luteum. In males, the hormone is often called interstitial cell stimulating hormone (ICSH) because it acts primarily by stimulating the interstitial Leydig cells in the testis to secrete testosterone.

7. Follicle-stimulating hormone FSH

This gonadotrophic hormone is a glycoprotein hormone also synthesized and stored within particular basophilic cells in the adenohypophysis. In females its primary function is to stimulate the follicular development of the ovary. In males it stimulates spermatogenesis.

The two gonadotrophins (LH and FSH) are discussed in greater detail in Chapter 5.

The neurohypophysis and neurohypophysial hormones

Anatomy, histology, and development

The neurohypophysis consists of the supraoptic and paraventricular nuclei in the hypothalamus, the tracts of nerve fibres from the cell bodies in the hypothalamic nuclei, and the posterior lobe of the hypophysis (which contains most of the nerve terminals). The term is sometimes used to differentiate the posterior lobe of the hypophysis from the anterior lobe (the adenohypophysis), although functionally this is incorrect. A small percentage of nerve fibres terminate in the hypothalamic median eminence region (see Fig. 2.3).

Along the nerve fibres, small swellings called Herring bodies can be seen. Interspersed between the nerve fibres in the posterior pituitary are numerous glial cells called pituicytes.

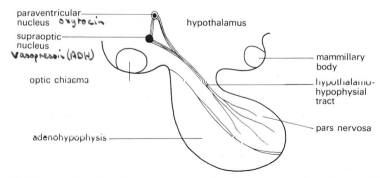

Fig.2.3 Diagram illustrating the various components of the neurohypophysis (the two hypothalamic nuclei, the hypothalamo-hypophysial nerve tract and the pars nervosa of the hypophysis).

The neurohypophysis develops from the infundibulum which grows from the hypothalamus in the floor of the forebrain. It receives its arterial bloodsupply from two main sources, the superior hypophysial artery in the median eminence region, and the inferior hypophysial artery in the lower part of the posterior lobe of the pituitary. An extensive capillary network is fairly regularly distributed throughout the posterior lobe of the hypophysis; the blood flows into veins which ultimately drain into the jugular veins.

The neurohypophysial hormones

Synthesis, storage, and release

The cell bodies of the supraoptic and paraventricular nuclei synthesize and secrete either one of two hormones, vasopressin or oxytocin. It is generally believed that vasopressin is synthesized mainly in the supraoptic nuclei while oxytocin is produced in the paraventricular nuclei. Each cell body synthesizes either vasopressin or oxytocin (one neurone—one hormone). Both these substances are octapeptides with similar chemical structures. Two forms of vasopressin have been identified in mammals; one contains the amino acid arginine, is called arginine vasopressin (AVP), and is found in most mammals including man, while the other contains the amino acid lysine, is called lysine vasopressin (LVP), and is present in the pig and hippopotamus. The structures of both vasopressins are otherwise identical and include the amino acid phenylalanine.

Oxytocin differs from the two vasopressins by having the amino acids leucine instead of either arginine or lysine, and isoleucine instead of phenylalanine (see Fig. 2.4).

Following their synthesis, both oxytocin and vasopressin become associated with specific proteins called neurophysins which are also synthesized in the cell bodies. These molecular complexes become incorporated into granules which then migrate down the nerve axons at a rate of 1–2 mm per day as a result of axoplasmic flow (axonal transport). The granules collect at the nerve terminals and also, apparently, in the Herring bodies along the nerve axons which may act as storage sites. The nerve endings are intimately related to the capillaries

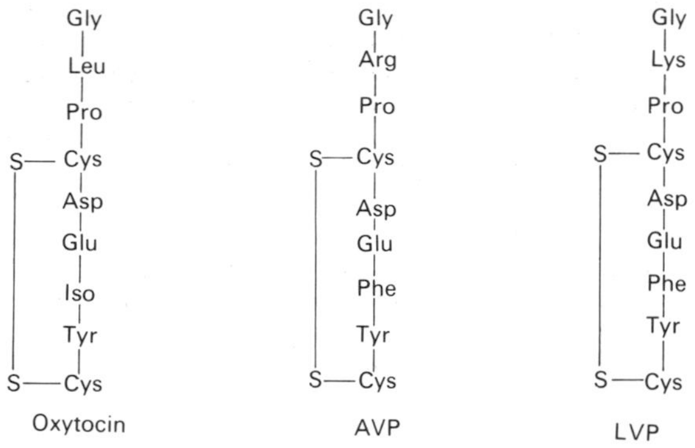

```
      Gly                    Gly                    Gly
       |                      |                      |
      Leu                    Arg                    Lys
       |                      |                      |
      Pro                    Pro                    Pro
       |                      |                      |
  S— Cys              S—Cys              S— Cys
       |                      |                      |
      Asp                    Asp                    Asp
       |                      |                      |
      Glu                    Glu                    Glu
       |                      |                      |
      Iso                    Phe                    Phe
       |                      |                      |
      Tyr                    Tyr                    Tyr
       |                      |                      |
  S—Cys              S—Cys              S—Cys

    Oxytocin                AVP                    LVP
```

Fig.2.4   The chemical structures of oxytocin, arginine vasopressin (AVP), and lysine vasopressin (LVP). (The two cysteine amino acids are generally considered together as one amino acid, cystine.)

in the posterior lobe of the pituitary. Release of the neurohypophysial hormones is associated with the arrival of action potentials at the nerve endings which depolarize the terminal membranes. The granular contents are believed to be released into the blood-stream by reverse pinocytosis. Dissociation between neurohypophysial hormone and neurophysin protein is believed to occur during the releasing process. The neurophysins may simply serve as a storage system for oxytocin and vasopressin within the nerve axons. They may also act to protect the hormones from immediate axoplasmic proteolysis. Nevertheless they are believed to be released with the neurohypophysial hormones since they can be detected in the blood, although they probably do not bind the hormones once in the blood-stream.

1. Vasopressin

Actions
The principal physiological action of vasopressin is to stimulate the reabsorption of water from the tubular fluid in the collecting ducts of the renal nephrons. The blood-level of the hormone therefore directly determines the water balance of the body, and indirectly the concentration of osmotically active solutes in the extracellular fluid (ECF), the most important solute being sodium. As the main action of vasopressin is to increase the volume of water reabsorbed from the nephrons, it determines urinary concentration. In the presence of vasopressin, the urine excreted by the kidneys is concentrated and is associated with a fall in urine volume (antidiuresis); hence this hormone is commonly referred to as anti-diuretic hormone (ADH). The mechanism of action for vasopressin in the collecting ducts is apparently mediated by an increase in the intracellular cyclic AMP concentration, although the precise mechanism by which this substance increases permeability to water is unknown.

The term vasopressin denotes an action on blood-pressure, but while this effect was the first to be shown for this hormone it is not its main physiological action. Nevertheless if vasopressin is released in sufficient quantities from the neurohypophysis, it induces a generalized vasoconstriction which results in increased peripheral resistance leading to a rise in arterial blood-pressure. While small decrements of blood volume may stimulate vasopressin release, only substantial decreases (of the order of 10 per cent) induce a sufficient rise in the concentration of vasopressin in the blood for the vasopressor effect to be evident. Vasopressin may play an important role in maintaining arterial blood pressure in haemorrhage involving the loss of 500 ml of blood or more.

Vasoconstriction of uterine smooth muscle and myoepithelial cells of the breast can also be induced by large amounts of circulating vasopressin, and thus this hormone has some intrinsic oxytocic activity. Similarly, oxytocin when present in large quantities in the blood has intrinsic antidiuretic activity.

Control of release

The principal mechanism involved in the release of vasopressin is a variation of the plasma osmolality. As a change of hydration commonly leads to an alteration in the concentration of osmotically active solutes in the extracellular fluid (ECF), this mechanism ensures the maintenance of water balance and indirectly the concentration of these solutes. For example, an increase in plasma osmolality results in an increased release of vasopressin from the neurohypophysis. The change in plasma osmolality is detected by certain specialized cells believed to lie in close proximity to the cell bodies of the supraoptic nuclei in the hypothalamus although they may be the cell bodies themselves. These cells are called osmo-receptors, and in response to a hypertonic ECF they shrink and the number of action potentials increases. The increased osmo-receptor activity stimulates the supraoptic neurones which then release increased quantities of vasopressin from their nerve-endings; more water is reabsorbed from the nephrons and consequently the plasma tonicity falls. Following this decrease in the plasma osmolality (hypotonicity) the frequency of the discharge of action potentials from the osmo-receptors decreases and the stimulus for the release of vasopressin from the neurohypophysis is reduced.

A second mechanism involved in the control of vasopressin release concerns changes in blood-volume. The stimulus for the release of vasopressin in haemorrhage is the decrease in the stretch of certain pressure receptors, called volume-receptors. These are situated in the two atria, especially the left atrium (low-pressure receptors), and also in other parts of the cardiovascular system, particularly the baro-receptors (high-pressure receptors) in the carotid sinus and aortic arch. A fall of blood-volume results in a decrease in the number of action potentials from these pressure receptors. This fall in frequency stimulates the release of vasopressin by decreasing the tonic inhibitory effect normally induced by the volume and pressure receptors. An increased stimulation of these receptors, following volume expansion for example, increases the inhibition on the supraoptic cell bodies; consequently the release of vasopressin from the neurohypophysis is reduced. The higher centres of the brain are also able to exert a profound influence over neurohypophysial hormone release through an undefined adrenergic nerve pathway. Stimuli such as emotional or surgical stresses probably cause the release of vasopressin through this pathway (see Fig. 2.5).

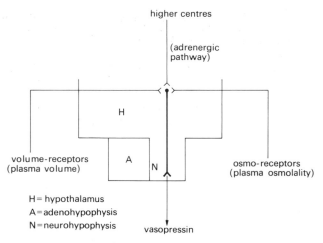

Fig.2.5 Diagram illustrating the principal control mechanisms involved in the release of vasopressin.

2. Oxytocin

Actions

Oxytocin, which is present in the neurohypophysis of both males and females, exerts its known physiological effects only in females. Oxytocin stimulates the contraction of the smooth muscle of the uterus and the lactating mammary glands. Contraction of the uterus in response to oxytocin is only observed during the late stages of pregnancy when oestrogens are secreted in increasing quantities relative to the concentration of circulating progestagens. It is believed that depolarization of uterine smooth muscle membranes by oxytocin occurs under the influence of oestrogens which 'prepare' the uterus for parturition by decreasing the resting potentials. Progestagens are believed to inhibit the action of oxytocin by increasing the resting membrane potential. While it may be that oxytocin plays a part in parturition, it is generally accepted that the mechanism of induction of labour is still uncertain. Oxytocin has been shown to be a useful therapeutic agent in inducing labour, but the physiological importance of this action and the mechanism whereby it induces uterine contractions remain obscure (see Chapter 5). Oxytocin if administered in large amounts, for instance to initiate the onset of labour, can have an antidiuretic effect. Oxytocin is necessary for the contraction of the myoepithelial cells of the milk ducts in the lactating mammary glands. Consequently, milk is ejected from the breasts when an appropriate stimulus (e.g. suckling) is applied, and this is known as the milk ejection reflex.

Control of release

Oxytocin release is stimulated in the lactating mother by suckling. Tactile receptors in the breasts, especially round the nipples, when stimulated initiate action potentials which propagate along afferent nerve fibres through the spinal cord and midbrain to the hypothalamus. The cell bodies in the paraventricular nucleus are then stimulated, resulting in the release of oxytocin. It is believed that other receptors in the uterus, and possibly in the mucosal walls of the vagina respond to stretch and initiate action potentials in afferent nerve fibres which ultimately stimulate the release of oxytocin from the neurohypophysis. The influence of other parts of the brain on the release of oxytocin, such as an emotional stress inhibiting lactation, is well documented. In general vasopressin and oxytocin are released independently, but they may occur together in some instances.

CLINICAL DISORDERS OF THE ADENOHYPOPHYSIS

Hormonal disturbances of the adenohypophysis are frequently the result of tumours in the region of this gland, and these are discussed in this chapter. The adenohypophysis secretes at least six different hormones and the various endocrine disturbances can be considered as excess of deficiency conditions for each individual hormone. In practice, a single adenohypophysial hormone deficiency is quite rare, and it is more common to find that the secretions of several hormones from the adenohypophysis are affected together. However in the future, with the development of tests which can identify specific substances, single adenohypophysial hormone deficiencies may become more commonly apparent. Panhypopituitarism (Simmond's disease), a deficiency of all the adenohypophysial hormones, is considered separately. Since the investigations to be followed for many of these conditions are often identical, they are considered first.

Investigations

1. Measurements of the appropriate hormone concentration in the plasma and, if possible, the quantities excreted in the urine in 24 hours. Tests may be employed to either stimulate or depress the levels of trophic hormone (see Chapter 12).

2. *Measurements of the concentrations of hormone secreted by the target endocrine glands* in the plasma and urine (see Chapter 12).

3. The *visual fields* are determined.

4. *Radiography of the skull.* Tumours in this region may induce general changes, namely:
   a. a double floor of the fossa, although claimed to be a common and normal finding, can nevertheless indicate the possibility of a tumour being present;
   b. distortion of the sella turcica;
   c. alterations in the vault of the skull, if the intracranial pressure has been raised for a long period.

Specific changes may also be seen: erosion of the anterior and/or posterior clinoids; calcification may occur with craniopharyngioma. In acromegaly (excess somatotrophin release in the adult) not only may there be an enlargement of the sella but also thickening of the skull, enlargement of the paranasal sinuses and widening of the mandibular angle.

5. While radiography may only suggest the possibility of an abnormality this may be resolved by *tomography*. Computerized axial tomography (EMI scan) provides a more accurate picture, but unfortunately it is only of value if there is suprasellar extension.

6. *Radiography of particular areas* in specific hormonal disorders:
   a. In 'pituitary' dwarfism radiography of the wrists will reveal any alteration of bone age in relation to chronological age.
   b. Radiography of the hands in acromegaly reveals not only the characteristic 'tufting' of the terminal phalanges, but also an increase of the soft tissue.

Tumours

Tumours of the adenohypophysis are a rare cause of intracranial neoplasms (about 10 per cent). Adenohypophysial tumours classically have been separated into three groups: chromophobe, eosinophil, or basophil, depending on the cell type affected. Since a mixture of cells may sometimes be affected, a classification based on the particular hormone secretion which is disturbed may be preferable. More sophisticated classifications have been applied, based on specialized histological staining techniques, but these are complex and even confusing. However, provided the limitation of the classical separation is appreciated it can still be applied, and for simplicity is adopted in this book.

A chromophobe adenoma may become very large, expanding the sella turcica, and even extending beyond the fossa. The eosinophil variety may expand the sella; frequently the so-called eosinophil adenoma is a mixture of chromophobe and eosinophil cells. Basophil adenomas are small and rarely distort the sella turcica.

Craniopharyngioma occurs in a remnant of the embryonic growth of ectoderm from the mouth. It occurs in the sella or more commonly in the suprasellar region and it usually develops in the young (5–10 years). Whether intrasellar compression of the adenohypophysis occurs depends on the position of the craniopharyngioma. In the suprasellar position the hypothalamus is damaged and may result in diabetes insipidus, obesity, or other hypothalamic disturbances.

Symptoms induced by any of these tumours may be due to pressure effects; for example headache is a common complaint, while disturbance of vision is due to lesions impinging on the optic nerve or chiasma. The typical bitemporal hemianopia may not be noticed by the patient, and is only detected when determining the visual fields; initially the defect may not be symmetrical. Ophthalmoscopy, which forms an essential part of any neurological examination, may reveal optic atrophy, resulting from compression of the optic nerves by the tumour (papilloedema is rare). It is uncommon for adenohypophysial tumours to involve other cranial nerves, but, when they do, those affected are the first, third, fourth, and sixth nerves.

Individual hormonal disturbances

In the past it was accepted that adenohypophysial malfunction was a fault within the gland itself, but now it is possible that in some conditions the disorder is of hypothalamic origin. Certainly, an isolated gonadotrophic condition associated with an olfactory defect (Kallman's syndrome) is now accepted as being of hypothalamic origin. In these patients FSH/LHRH is apparently absent and they can be treated successfully (if young) with hormone replacement therapy. An isolated deficiency of growth hormone in children may also be due to a hypothalamic disorder. It is generally accepted that hyperprolactinaemia (excluding the drug-induced variety) is a consequence of a failure of the hypothalamus to secrete normal quantities of the inhibitor factor (PIF).

1. Gonadotrophin

Excess

Sexual precocity associated with increased gonadotrophin secretion is usually induced by cerebral tumours in the region of the hypothalamus (occasionally aberrant pinealomata) in which case there are often changes associated with hypothalamic disorders such as diabetes insipidus and obesity. This is considered in greater detail in Chapter 5.

Deficiency

This is the first trophic hormone to be affected in lesions of the adenohypophysis. If it occurs in the young, the child is often (but not invariably) tall for its age and the accessory sex organs and secondary sex characteristics fail to develop. Isolated gonadotrophic defects may be familial, sometimes occurring with anosmia or defects of smell (Kallman's syndrome), or with congenital defects such as cleft palate, hair-lip, and facial asymmetry. If the condition occurs in the adult the secondary sex characteristics show evidence of atrophy, and there is scanty or absent pubic and axillary hair, infertility, and the possible loss of libido. In the young female, amenorrhoea and some atrophy of the external genitalia and vagina occurs. In the male, facial hair growth diminishes, but marked changes in the size of the testes and penis are not usual. There may be a defect of LH alone in the male in which case reference is sometimes made to the 'fertile eunuch'. Spermatogenesis is normal, indicating that enough LH (interstitial cell stimulating hormone, ICSH) is secreted to allow for sufficient testosterone production. It may be that the testosterone only acts locally so that while there is sufficient hormone release for the development of the spermatozoa, this is insufficient for the development of the male accessory sex organs and secondary sex characteristics. Thus the patients are eunuchoid and commonly have gynaecomastia. The testes are usually of normal size. A deficiency of FSH alone has, as yet, to be described.

TREATMENT: At present therapy with FSH/LHRH appears to be very successful, and could well become the therapy of choice. Gonadotrophins have hitherto been advocated, the source of LH being pregnant women's urine while FSH is derived from the urine of post-menopausal women, which also contains some LH. It is probably advisable to start with LH 2000 to 4000 IU thrice weekly. In males serum testosterone levels will determine when the dose is adequate. The interstitial cells of Leydig should begin to mature and the seminiferous tubules will then develop as a result of the stimulating action of testosterone. Should spermatogenesis not develop satisfactorily FSH is also given (150 IU thrice weekly). When full sexual development has been achieved the treatment should be altered to testosterone which may be given sublingually (10–40 mg daily of Testoral), or monthly by intramuscular injections of Sustenon 250 mg. Occasionally testosterone by itself without prior treatment with gonadotrophins may induce spermatogenesis. Although replacement therapy with trophic hormones has been advocated in the past, it is both time-consuming and costly. Furthermore, while it may be possible to induce puberty and sometimes to initiate spermatogenesis, the patient usually remains infertile, although an occasional success has been claimed. Testosterone is cheap, easy to administer, and will induce growth of accessory sex organs and characteristics if therapy is commenced in the young, but they will remain infertile. Testosterone levels are raised directly (or indirectly) to normal adult levels. The epiphyses of the long bones will be stimulated (unless they have fused already) until fusion occurs. There is thus an initial spurt of growth before growth cessation.

If the deficiency develops in an adult woman, restoration of fertility is possible, hence the claim that gonadotrophin replacement therapy is justified. It appears possible that in the future the ideal therapy may be LHRH.

2. Prolactin

Excess

It is now accepted that hyperprolactinaemia will suppress gonadal function. In women, amenorrhoea and infertility and sometimes galactorrhoea (see Plate 2.1) may occur. Hyperprolactinaemia in men is a cause of infertility associated with a loss of libido.

Excess prolactin secretion may be due to micro-adenomata of the adenohypophysis. This is of particular relevance with respect to the woman in whom fertility has been successfully restored with bromocriptine, because during pregnancy and after parturition there is frequently a dramatic enlargement of these microadenomata.

Hyperprolactinaemia has also been suggested as a cause of (a) premenstrual tension, (b) idiopathic oedema, (c) migraine, (d) continued fluid retention seen in heart failure or in conditions in which there is oedema, (e) eclampsia. It is claimed that the failure to respond to bromocriptine in these conditions may be due to the administration of an insufficiently high dose of drug.

Hyperprolactinaemia may also be induced by drugs such as oral contraceptives, metoclopramide, methyl dopa, antidepressants, and tranquillizers; this hormonal disturbance may continue even after cessation of therapy. Hyperprolactinaemia may also occur in myxoedema, in adrenal and in hepatic failure. It may very occasionally occur in patients with ectopic secretion of the hormone from a carcinoma of the bronchus.

TREATMENT: When the hyperprolactinaemia is believed to be of adenohypo-

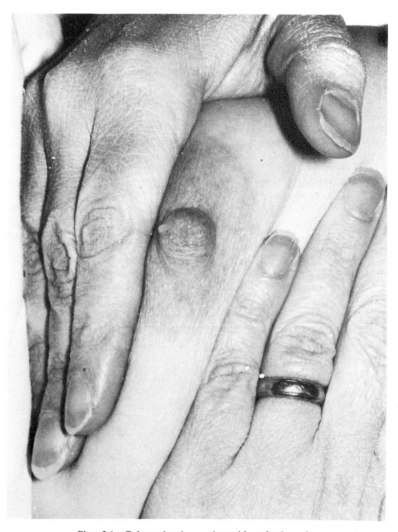

Plate 2.1   Galactorrhea in a patient with prolactinaemia.

physial origin, bromocriptine is used; the details are given in the section on acromegaly, but a smaller dose is used, as these patients appear to be more prone to the adverse effects of the drug. If a tumour is found, surgery or radiotherapy is advocated (see acromegaly).

If there is the possibility of microadenomata in a patient who is being treated for infertility, it may be advisable to apply appropriate radiation therapy to the sella turcica region during pregnancy.

Deficiency

This occurs with other adenohypophysial deficiencies and the only known clinical effect is the inhibition of lactation in post-puerperal women. There are other causes for failure of lactation, but the possibility of Sheehan's disease (p. 30) must always be considered.

3. Somatotrophin (growth hormone)

Excess

Excessive secretion of somatotrophin is usually due to an eosinophil adenoma of the adenohypophysis. The incidence of eosinophil tumours is second to the much larger group of chromophobe adenomata. If it occurs in a child gigantism is produced; growth is accelerated and heights in excess of 1·5 m (8 ft) may be reached. It is claimed that initially muscular strength is increased in gigantism, but this is soon replaced by weakness. If the condition continues unabated after maturity is reached, the changes of acromegaly are seen. Acromegaly is the name given to the characteristic clinical appearance of patients who in adulthood develop an oversecretion of somatotrophin. The general appearance of a typical, fully developed acromegalic is that of a large, burly individual—if the patient is a male the features are reminiscent of a pugilist. There is general coarsening of the facial features due to an increase of connective tissue, for example thickening of the lips. Increased cartilaginous growth results in an enlargement of the ears and nose. The growth of the mandible leads to a jutting jaw (prognathism), and alveolar bone growth causes the teeth to separate (see Plates 2.2, 2.3, and 2.4). The enlargement of the frontal and maxillary sinuses

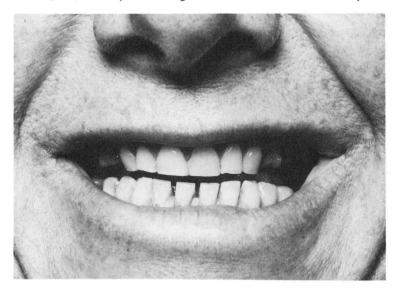

Plate 2.2   The separation of the teeth due to the growth of alveolar bone in a patient with acromegaly.

results in a prominent brow and a long face. In addition to these facial changes there is the well-recognized broadening and enlargement of the hands and feet due to periosteal overgrowth, and thickening of the connective tissue. The cartilaginous overgrowth of the ribs results in thickening of the costal margins; there is a marked kyphosis (increased curvature of the vertebrae). The tongue is enlarged and usually there is a generalized enlargement of the internal organs such as the spleen, liver, kidneys, and almost invariably the heart. In addition, the blood-pressure may be elevated.

In the florid case just described the diagnosis is obvious, but it must be realized that the disease follows an insidious course. It is therefore important to be aware of the possibility of the diagnosis in any patient whose features have become coarser, particularly if the patient notices that the sizes of gloves and shoes have increased. Usually there are warning symptoms such as joint pains, excessive sweating, and paraesthesiae of the hands and feet some 10–15 years before the typical changes have appeared. Headaches are not always a presenting feature.

The facial appearance may superficially resemble that of myxoedema, possibly because in the latter condition there is also an enlargement of the tongue, and the voice is husky. This confusion of diseases can be avoided by a detailed inspection.

Acromegaly may present as a fulminant variety in which death may occur within a few years, or, somewhat infrequently, the disease may suddenly cease to progress. It is important to note that even though there may be no further physical change in some patients the levels of somatotrophin may remain high. In those patients with raised blood levels of the hormone (the majority) the

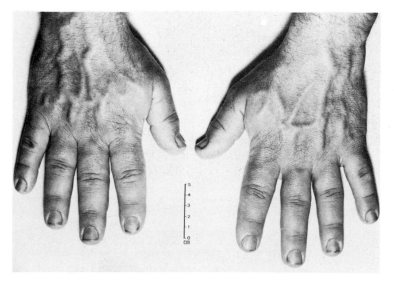

Plate 2.3   The characteristic broadening and enlargement of the fingers due to the increased periosteal growth and thickening of connective tissue in a patient with acromegaly.

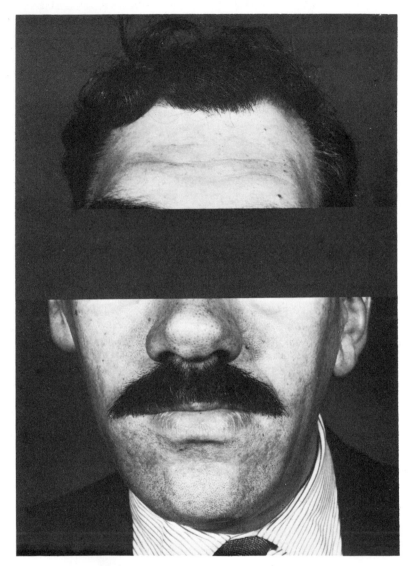

Plate 2.4   A male patient with acromegaly, clearly showing the general coarsening of the facial features (e.g. the lips) due to the increased growth of connective tissue, and the enlargement of the ears and nose due to increased growth of cartilage. The prominent brow and the lengthening of the face can also be seen.

disease will progress, and treatment is essential as death may commonly occur due to cardiovascular disease, or to adrenal failure caused by hypopituitarism following a haemorrhage into the tumour, or to the complications of diabetes mellitus.

ASSOCIATED ENDOCRINE DISORDERS: Most patients have slightly elevated prolactin levels, and occasionally galactorrhoea which can only be detected by compression of the breasts; sometimes spontaneous lactation may occur in women. About 25 per cent of the patients have impaired carbohydrate tolerance with symptomless glycosuria, but only half of these have overt diabetes mellitus. While the basal metabolic rate may be raised, hyperthyroidism is rare; if myxoedema occurs this usually follows the destruction of the adenohypophysis. Hypogonadism may occur resulting in reduced libido, impotence, gynaecomastia and in females oligo- or amenorrhoea. Occasionally diabetes insipidus may be present due to the tumour impinging on the relevant hypothalamic area. Multiple endocrine adenomatosis is a rare condition in which enlargement of the parathyroids and islets of Langerhans occur together with acromegaly (see Chapter 9).

TREATMENT: Any patient with a raised plasma level of somatotrophin must be treated. If there is radiological evidence of expansion of the sella or involvement of the optic nerves (and chiasma) or raised intracranial pressure it is generally agreed that treatment must be directed towards the adenohypophysis itself. In the less severe conditions drug therapy or radiotherapy may be sufficient; otherwise surgery is advocated.

(a) Bromocriptine (dopamine agonist). If the tumour is not producing local intracranial effects, the treatment of choice is bromocriptine. In acromegalic patients an important complication of bromocriptine therapy is gastric haemorrhage. To reduce the side-effects of the drug (nausea, vomiting and postural hypotension) the initial dose is 1·25 mg with the evening meal. The dose is increased every 3–4 days reaching the full dose of 20 mg/day (5 mg four times a day with food) in 3–4 weeks. The regression of the connective tissue during this therapy is remarkable. However, it is essential to assess repeatedly the size of the sella turcica by radiography to ensure that there is no evidence of expansion.

(b) Radiation (external high voltage) giving a total course of 45 by (4500 rad).

(c) Radioactive implants: at present the one of choice is yttrium-90. However, with this therapy there is the marked disadvantage of subsequent cerebrospinal rhinorrhoea.

(d) Surgery: total or partial removal of the adenohypophysis is performed if there are local symptoms such as ocular palsies and raised intracranial pressure.

Deficiency

Hormones do not appear to play a significant role in the growth of the fetus and a deficiency of somatotrophin at this stage does not affect the birthweight. It is therefore only after birth that there is an impairment of growth, and hence the condition is not usually recognized until after the first year of life.

CLINICAL FEATURES: The parents usually bring their affected child for examination because of a failure to grow. The child has an immature face, and is short for its age; skeletal immaturity is not marked, but there is progressive physical retardation (dwarfism). A deficiency of this hormone is not a common cause of a failure to grow. It is difficult to define normal growth-rate without referring to a growth chart (e.g. Tanner–Whitehouse chart). It is then possible

Table 2.2   Diagnosis of important varieties of short stature

	Constitutional delay in growth and adolescence	Familial short stature	Pituitary dwarfism	Hypothyroid dwarfism	Turner's syndrome
Family history	Positive	Positive	Usually negative	Negative	Usually negative
Birth weight and height	Normal	Reduced	Normal	Normal	Slightly reduced
Pattern of growth	Rather slow from birth	Slow from birth	Slow from few months after birth	Slow from birth	Slow from birth
Epiphyseal development	Moderate but not progressive retardation	Almost normal	Progressive retardation	Marked retardation	Within normal but wide variation
Features	Immature but later normal	Mature	Immature	Infantile	Often characteristic
Puberty	Late but eventually normal	Normal	Usually delayed unless solitary growth hormone deficiency	Delayed	Usually no signs except in mosaics
Serum cholesterol	Normal	Normal	Raised	Raised	Normal
Growth hormone level	Normal	Normal	Low	Normal	Normal
Gonadotrophin level (after puberty)	Normal	Normal	Low unless solitary growth hormone deficiency	Normal or may be raised	Raised

Reproduced from Hall, Anderson, Smart, and Besser (1974): *Fundamentals of clinical endocrinology* (second edition) by courtesy of the authors and Pitman Medical Publishing Company Ltd.

to determine whether the short child grows at a rate parallel to normal in which case the cause is usually 'constitutional'.

The 'pituitary' dwarf can be distinguished from other causes of short stature by examination of the various characteristics which are given in Table 2.2. In addition there may be gonadotrophic deficiencies and, less frequently, corticotrophin and TSH deficiencies. Clinically these deficiencies are seen as an atrophy of the target organs. A similar condition of dwarfism may occur when the endogenous 'somatotrophin' is apparently inactive or when the target cells are insensitive to somatotrophin. It is important to remember that exogenous cortisone, if given in large enough doses in the young, inhibits growth; sufficient hormone may be absorbed from topical application to large areas of the skin. Besides a congenital deficiency of somatotrophin, secretion may be impaired due to a chromophobe adenoma, an eosinophilic granuloma, Hand--Schuller–Christian disease, or following healed tuberculosis meningitis.

TREATMENT: The ideal treatment is human somatotrophin. A dose as small as 2·5 mg twice weekly may be sufficient, but usually the quantity administered is 5–10 mg (subcutaneously) in addition to the hormonal replacement of any associated deficiencies.

4. Corticotrophin

Excess

The effects are due to enhanced quantities of cortisol and androgens from the adrenals. The resulting clinical picture which this induces (Cushing's syndrome) is considered in Chapter 4. Excluding iatrogenic causes, Cushing's syndrome in some 75 per cent of cases is due to excess production of corticotrophin (Cushing's disease) if ectopic secretion of corticotrophin (Chapter 9) is excluded.

TREATMENT: This is considered in Chapter 4.

Deficiency

Typically this is one of the last trophic hormones to be affected when adenohypophysial function is impaired. The clinical picture is essentially similar to the changes seen in Addison's disease (see Chapter 4), but there is no pigmentation and only a slight impairment of aldosterone secretion.

5. Thyrotrophin

Excess

In the past hyperthyroidism was always believed to be due to an excess secretion of thyrotrophin, but this view is no longer held. Indeed thyrotrophin secretion is markedly reduced in thyrotoxicosis. Only very rarely is thyrotoxicosis due to over secretion of adenohypophysial thyrotrophin and when it occurs it is usually associated with acromegaly.

TREATMENT: The underlying lesion is treated.

Deficiency

This induces hypothyroidism, and on occasion it may be difficult to differentiate from a primary defect of the thyroid gland. Usually there is evidence of other trophic hormone deficiencies resulting in, for example, gonadal deficiency which produces changes such as amenorrhoea in females, and scanty pubic and axillary hair in both sexes. The reader is referred to Chapter 6 for further details on hypothyroidism.

TREATMENT: Thyroxine is given as for myxoedema, in addition to cortisol 10 mg three times a day.

Hypopituitarism

Hypopituitarism produces its effect by inducing secondary atrophy of the gonads, thyroid, and adrenals. Changes are not present until some 75 per cent of the adenohypophysis is destroyed. The hypopituitarism which may occur after parturition (post-partum necrosis) is called Sheehan's disease. In panhypopituitarism the hormones are usually affected in the following order: gonadotrophin, prolactin, somatotrophin, TSH, and ACTH. Total absence of all these hormones is not compatible with life. In an adult, destruction of the adenohypophysis may be due to a chromophobe adenoma, infarction of a tumour, post-partum necrosis, surgical removal, destruction by radiation, or rarely to a secondary deposit from a malignant tumour. Adenohypophysial deficiency in children is usually due to a craniopharyngioma, and this will result in dwarfism as well as other hormonal deficiencies.

The reader should refer to the relevant trophic hormone deficiencies (e.g. pp. 21–30).

The acute form can present with nausea, vomiting, weakness, and hypotension. The clinical features may resemble that of an Addisonian crisis, but there is little disturbance of the plasma electrolytes. Sometimes these patients have markedly elevated temperatures (see Chapter 11). The chronic form of adenohypophysial insufficiency is more frequently seen. Patients with adenohypophysial insufficiency may lose weight, but this is rarely marked, and the idea that cachexia is common in this condition should be discarded. The skin has a characteristic pallid or waxen appearance, which is due to depigmentation, the capacity to tan in ultraviolet light being impaired. While there is an anaemia, this is usually mild and would not be responsible for the pallor. It is important to remember that these patients have a poor response to stress. While there is the expected increase in insulin sensitivity, the patient may only occasionally suffer hypoglycaemic attacks. Hyponatraemia is common, but this is due to the water retention which may result from adrenal deficiency possibly by a reduction in glomerular filtration rate (GFR), or by an enhancement of the response by the renal tubules to vasopressin or to increased plasma levels of this hormone (the mechanism is unknown), or to a combination of these factors. The adenohypophysial deficiencies which occur have been discussed under the relevant sections.

TREATMENT: If possible the cause of the deficiency, such as an adenoma, should be removed but unfortunately adenohypophysial deficiency usually persists after the surgical procedure. The subsequent treatment in the adult is systematic, replacing the thyroid hormone deficiency and if necessary supplementing this with cortisol. As hypothyroidism can, on clinical examination, be confused with hypopituitarism it is probably wise to give the steroid before the thyroxine. Thyroxine therapy must be commenced at a low dose (0·05 mg daily). Androgen administration to men will increase their general strength and may restore their potency. In women it may be possible to restore fertility by following the treatment described on p. 97. With full hormonal replacement therapy the clinical response is highly satisfactory to the patient and the doctor.

CLINICAL DISORDERS OF THE NEUROHYPOPHYSIS

Tumours of the pars nervosa are very rare and when they occur consist of nervous tissue. The main clinical interest in this gland are the disorders known as diabetes insipidus which results from a relative or absolute deficiency of arginine vasopressin (AVP) and the 'syndrome of inappropriate secretion' of the hormone. This syndrome should not be confused with the ectopic secretion of the hormone (Chapter 9).

Individual hormone disorders

Arginine vasopressin

In this section reference will be made to antidiuretic hormone (ADH) instead of arginine vasopressin (AVP), as this is the usual clinical term.

Excess

As yet there has been no reported case of excess AVP secretion by a tumour of the pars nervosa. An excessive secretion however may occur in a wide variety of clinical conditions—syndrome of 'inappropriate' secretion of ADH; these are summarized in the Table 2.3. It is assumed that this syndrome exists if the following are present; hyponatraemia, urine osmolality in excess of that of plasma, an adequate osmolar excretion, normal skin turgor, and normal renal and adrenal function. Recently the syndrome has been defined such that its occurrence is accepted when 'the amount of ADH released and the elevation of urine osmolality which it produces are considered to be inappropriate only in relationship to the level of plasma osmolality or serum sodium concentration'.

Clinically, reference is often made to this syndrome if there is hyponatraemia, indirect evidence of an excess of ADH, and no evidence of change of extracellular fluid (ECF) volume. However, the diagnosis must depend on an absolute increase of ADH or on proof that the level is higher than that which one would expect with regard to the diagnosis of hyponatraemia.

Table 2.3 Conditions in which the 'syndrome of inappropriate secretion of ADH (AVP)†' is reported to occur, excluding 'ectopic secretion'

Central nervous system disease Meningitis and encephalitis Head injury Brain tumour and abscess Subarachnoid and subdural haemorrhage Cerebrovascular thrombosis Guillain–Barre syndrome Acute intermittent porphyria (with 　cerebral involvement) *Pulmonary disease* Pneumonia, especially 　bronchopneumonia in the elderly Tuberculosis Cavitation (e.g. aspergillosis)	*Endocrine disease* Hypoadrenalism Hypopituitarism Hypothyroidism *Miscellaneous* Post-operative Drugs, e.g. Clofibrate (ethyl 　chlorophenoxyisobutyrate) Hepatic cirrhosis *'Idiopathic'*

† or similar antidiuretic peptide.
The conditions listed on this table are somewhat arbitrarily selected, as there is some diversity of opinion on the definition of this syndrome. For example, 'post-operative' is included under 'miscellaneous'. This condition could be regarded as one in which one would expect there to be an increase of ADH, as pain is an accepted physiological stimulus to the neurohypophysis.

CLINICAL FEATURES: Frequently, even though the hyponatraemia may be severe, symptoms are absent. There may be generalized weakness, malaise, poor mental function, anorexia and nausea- oedema is usually absent. If the concentration of sodium falls to 100–110 mmol/l, the temperature may be subnormal and the tendon reflexes sluggish: if the plasma sodium falls below about 100 mmol/l there may be an extensor plantar response. Any further fall results in some clouding of consciousness, epileptiform attacks, and eventually coma.

Hyponatraemia occurs in many conditions, and may be due to excess sodium loss due to gastrointestinal disturbance, salt-losing nephritis, adrenocortical deficiency, or oedematous states, for example congestive heart failure. True hyponatraemia must be differentiated from the apparent or pseudo hyponatraemia of hyperproteinaemia (e.g. myeloma) or of hyperlipidaemia (one litre of plasma is no longer approximately equal to one litre of water).

INVESTIGATIONS:

1. The plasma sodium concentration, plasma osmolality, and urine osmolality are estimated. These estimations are best employed if the blood is taken at about the midpoint of the period of the urine collection. Urine osmolality should exceed that of the plasma.

2. Standard tests are employed to assess adrenal and renal function. Water loads are employed to assess renal function, only if the plasma sodium is above 125 mmol/l.

3. Volume compartments of the body may be measured. Probably the volume

of total body water is the most reliable, as plasma volume and ECF volume are not invariably raised. In this syndrome urine osmolality exceeds that of plasma; renal and adrenal function are normal, and the total body water is raised.

4. If available, radioimmunoassay or bioassay measurements of AVP levels in blood or urine confirm the diagnosis.

TREATMENT: The underlying lesion must be treated or the offending drug removed. Water intake is restricted to 500–600 ml/24 h. Fludrocortisone, cortisone, or other corticosteroids should not be administered, as this will indirectly cause the retention of greater quantities of water without altering the plasma concentration of sodium. Similarly intravenous 'normal' saline will not significantly raise the plasma sodium and may be detrimental. Other drugs such as lithium or demoxycycline have been tried with little success.

Deficiency

Diabetes insipidus results from a relative or complete absence of ADH and is sometimes referred to as cranial diabetes insipidus in order to avoid confusion with nephrogenic diabetes insipidus which is believed to be due to insensitivity of the renal tubule to vasopressin. Probably the most common cause of diabetes insipidus is head injury or following surgical procedures in the vicinity of the hypophysis. Tumours, intrasellar and suprasellar (craniopharyngioma), and other causes, namely granulomatous infiltration, sarcoidosis, Hand--Schuller–Christian disease, and following healed tuberculous meningitis, give rise to diabetes insipidus only if the lesion involves the median eminence as well as the pars nervosa. No causal factor can be detected in approximately one-third of the patients presenting with diabetes insipidus, possibly because the disorder is due to an enzyme defect resulting in impaired hormone synthesis. This group in whom no causal factor can be determined is often referred to as primary, to distinguish it from those with a detectable lesion (secondary). Primary diabetes insipidus is divided into the idiopathic and familial. The former is by far the commoner and may occur at any age, but it rarely affects infants; whereas the familial type is found in relatives and may occur in infants.

CLINICAL FEATURES: There is an insatiable thirst and intense polyuria (up to 20 l per day). While the onset of these changes is usually gradual, it may sometimes be sudden and dramatic; the danger of dehydration in diabetes insipidus in adverse environmental conditions is a very real one. The same danger occurs in an unconscious patient following a head injury or intracranial surgery when full fluid replacement may not be maintained.

There are only two conditions which may be confused with diabetes insipidus, namely compulsive water drinking, and nephrogenic diabetes insipidus. While the term 'compulsive water drinker' implies a desire to drink water, these patients frequently prefer other fluids (e.g. Coca-cola), unlike patients with cranial diabetes insipidus who almost invariably prefer water.

INVESTIGATIONS:

1. Plasma urea and electrolytes and full blood-count show the expected changes of dehydration in diabetes insipidus.

2. The urine concentration in diabetes insipidus is usually of the order of 100 mosm/kg H_2O, rising to about 600–800 mosm/kg H_2O following an injection of vasopressin, whereas the patient with nephrogenic diabetes insipidus is unresponsive to the hormone. Vasopressin can be given intravenously as 100 mU bolus followed by 5 mU/min intravenously for 1 h. This method does require catheterization of the bladder allowing the urine to be collected as it is being excreted; hence a raised response can be detected. The intramuscular route is the simpler as catheterization is not required; 5 U of aqueous vasopressin or 2·5 U of vasopressin tanate in oil is given at about 1900 h. The bladder is emptied at bedtime and maximum urine osmolality is usually achieved at 12–16 h after the injection. Another method is to use the analogue 1-desamino-8-D-arginine vasopressin (DDAVP) intranasally. The major disadvantage of these tests is that in the compulsive water-drinker the procedure may be dangerous. It is therefore advisable to employ this test immediately after the water deprivation test and thus avoid water retention (see 3).

3. Dehydration by fluid restriction until the body weight is reduced by 3–5 per cent in the adult only results in a maximum osmolality in the region of 300–500/kg H_2O. This test must be carried out under very careful supervision.

The compulsive water-drinker when subjected to the same test shows greater increases in osmolality (800–1000 mosm/kg H_2O), but sometimes these patients are inexplicably unable to concentrate the urine. Hence the differential diagnosis between diabetes insipidus and the compulsive water-drinker may be difficult, in which case various further tests, varying in complexity, have to be used.

4. Tests of value also include the administration of a placebo instead of the hormone, the former being remarkably effective only in the compulsive water-drinker; these patients usually have a low plasma osmolality.

5. As the blood concentration of AVP in the normal state is at the lower limit of sensitivity for both bioassay and radioimmunoassay techniques, measurement of the plasma concentration in diabetes insipidus is still of little value.

TREATMENT: The recent development of DDAVP, an analogue of AVP which has a greater antidiuretic potency without the vasopressor side-effects, has simplified the treatment of diabetes insipidus. Therapy consists of administering 0·1–0·2 ml of DDAVP intranasally, once or twice daily. With the introduction of this therapy, diuretics, which were moderately effective by reducing the filtered load, and chlorpropamide are no longer employed in cranial diabetes insipidus. However, diuretic therapy (e.g. thiazides) are partially successful for nephrogenic diabetes insipidus.

Oxytocin

Excess

No clinical syndrome has been described due to an excess of the hormone.

Insufficiency

This usually occurs in association with lack of AVP (cranial diabetes insipidus). The absence of oxytocin does not appear to influence the first and second stages of labour, but it has been claimed that in this condition the third stage may be delayed. However, the defect does give rise to the inability of the mother to suckle her infant.

3 The adrenal medulla

PHYSIOLOGY

The adrenal medulla is the central part of the adrenal (suprarenal) gland which lies on the superior pole of the kidney. It secretes catecholamines of which in man 80 per cent consists of adrenalin (epinephrine), the remainder being noradrenalin (norepinephrine). The adrenal medullae are not essential for life since their function can be compensated for by increased sympathetic activity.

Anatomy, histology, and development

The adrenal medulla is embryologically derived from the neural crest, and consists of granule-containing cells which are called chromaffin cells. There is histological evidence to suggest that there are two types of cell, each synthesizing its specific hormone, adrenalin or noradrenalin. Approximately 80 per cent of the chromaffin cells in human adrenomedullary tissue appear to be of the type which synthesizes adrenalin.

The arterial blood-supply to the adrenal gland reaches the outer capsule of the gland from branches of the renal and phrenic arteries, although there is a less important arterial supply from the aorta. From the capillary plexus on the outer adrenal capsule most of the blood enters sinusoids which descend through the adrenal cortical tissue, perfusing the cells on the way. Thus most blood reaching the adrenal medulla is partly deoxygenated. There are also small medullary arteries which descend directly to the adrenal medulla from the outer capsule, and which provide a supply of true arterial blood. Venous blood drains via a central adrenal vein, which passes along the axis of the gland.

Functional significance of the adrenal medulla

The physiological importance of the adrenal medullae remains uncertain since they can be extirpated without any apparent deterioration in the general maintenance of homeostasis. Indeed, sensitivity of tissues to sympathetic nervous activity appears to increase in this situation. Nevertheless, the ability of the adrenal medullae to release catecholamines into the general circulation would suggest an important reinforcing mechanism which would not only prolong the direct effects of general sympathetic activity, but would also increase the blood concentration of energy substrates through the metabolic effects of circulating adrenalin. These metabolic effects are of particular relevance to the catecholamines since they emphasize the difference between a hormone such as adrenalin which can reach all cells of the body through the circulation, and noradrenalin which is released at nerve endings and acts on those cells with sympathetic innervations.

The release of catecholamines from the adrenal medulla as part of a general sympathetic stimulation is probably of particular importance in conditions of emergency and stress (the 'fear–fight–flight' situation first described by Cannon in 1920).

The catecholamines

Synthesis, storage, and release

The catecholamines (dopamine, noradrenalin, and adrenalin) are synthesized in the brain, at sympathetic postganglionic nerve endings, and at sites of chromaffin tissue such as the adrenal medullae. The synthetic pathway originates with the amino acid tyrosine (derived mainly from the diet, although hydroxylation of phenylaline in the liver is also important). Tyrosine is hydroxylated to L-dopa and this is then decarboxylated to dopamine, which is further hydroxylated to form noradrenalin (or norepinephrine). Noradrenalin can be converted to adrenalin (or epinephrine) by methylation, brought about by the enzyme phenylethanolamine-N-methyl transferase which is found only in adrenomedullary tissue, the organ of Zuckerkandl, and, in minute amounts, in the brain (see Fig. 3.1). Extremely high local concentrations of glucocorticoids from the adrenal cortex via the portal system are necessary for the methylation reaction in the adrenal medulla.

The catecholamines are stored in granules within the chromaffin cells of the adrenal medullae and their release is stimulated by acetylcholine from the preganglionic sympathetic nerve endings which innervate the chromaffin cells. The chromaffin cells may therefore be considered as specialized postganglionic sympathetic nerve fibres which can release their catecholamines directly into the blood-stream.

Direct electrical stimulation of certain areas in the hypothalamus which elicit general sympathetic discharge (with the release of catecholamines at the postganglionic sympathetic nerve endings for a local effect) also induces the release of catecholamines into the general circulation through stimulation of the adrenal medulla. In humans the principal catecholamine released from this gland is adrenalin, whereas at the postganglionic sympathetic nerve endings noradrenalin is released. It is interesting to note that direct electrical stimulation of selected parts of the hypothalamus associated with the release of catecholamines has been claimed to be selective with respect to the actual catecholamine released from the adrenal medulla; certain areas when stimulated, appear to be associated with the release of noradrenalin alone, whereas other areas appear to be related to the selective release of adrenalin. These observations indicate separate neuronal pathways relating the hypothalamus to the different cells in the adrenal medulla associated with the release of either one of the catecholamines from this endocrine gland.

Actions

The effects of adrenomedullary stimulation and sympathetic nerve stimulation are generally similar. There are, however, certain tissues in which adrenalin and noradrenalin produce different effects. The postulated existence of two different types of receptor, α and β, with different sensitivities for the various catecholamines would account for the different responses. According to this classification system, the α-receptors are sensitive to both adrenalin and noradrenalin; the β-receptors respond to adrenalin, but are in general relatively insensitive to noradrenalin. The various body systems which respond to adrenalin and/or noradrenalin are considered individually.

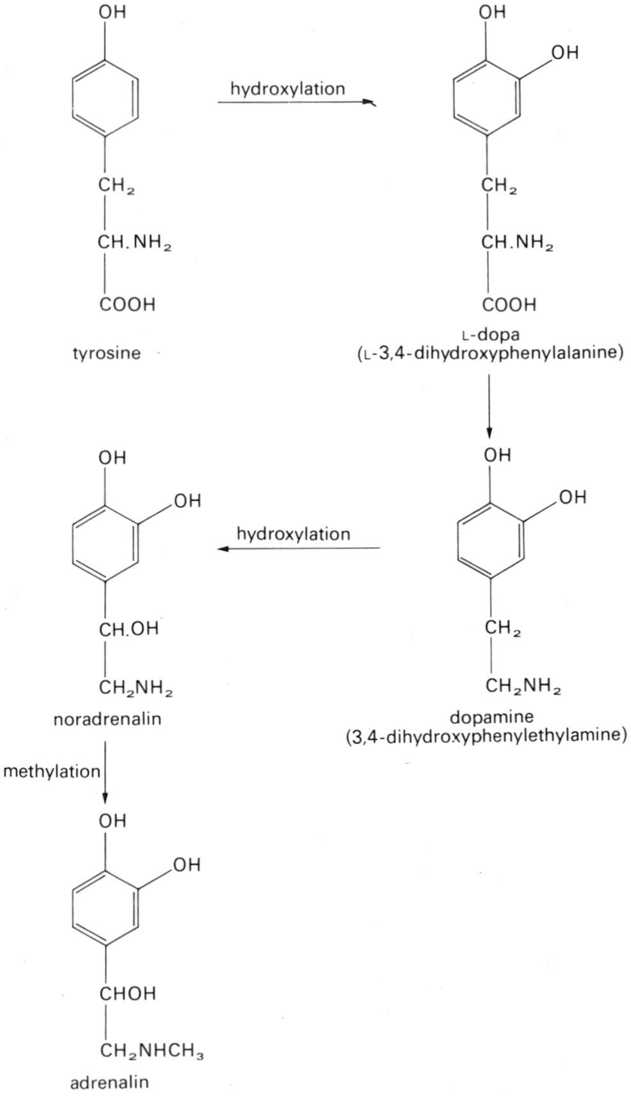

Fig.3.1 The principal features of the synthesis of noradrenalin and adrenalin.

1. Cardiovascular system

a. heart-rate: increased by both adrenalin and noradrenalin (positive chrono-tropic action);

b. force of contraction of heart muscle: increased by both adrenalin and noradrenalin (positive inotropic action);

c. coronary blood-flow: in man it is uncertain whether adrenalin or norad-renalin increase coronary blood-flow;

d. blood-vessels of skin, mucous membranes and splanchnic bed: vaso-constriction, by adrenalin and noradrenalin;

e. blood-vessels of skeletal muscle: vasoconstriction by noradrenalin, but chiefly vasodilatation by adrenalin.

As a result of the general vasoconstriction of blood vessels by noradrenaline, peripheral resistance to blood-flow is increased. This increase in peripheral resistance together with the increased stroke volume results in increased systolic and diastolic pressures such that the mean arterial blood-pressure rises. An increased mean arterial blood-pressure following the administration of noradrenalin stimulates the baro-receptors in the carotid sinus and aortic arch. The receptors in turn stimulate the medullary cardio-inhibitory centre which then reflexly inhibits the heart-rate through the vagus, overcoming the initial tachycardia. The actions of adrenalin on the heart are such that the systolic pressure increases and the diastolic pressure may decrease; the mean arterial blood-pressure following the administration of adrenalin therefore may not change, or if it does then only by increasing slightly. Since this catecholamine induces a vasodilatation in skeletal muscle, its vasoconstrictor effect on the blood-vessels of the skin and splanchnic bed is counteracted; the peripheral resistance therefore actually decreases, but the diastolic pressure may not fall because the stroke volume is increased. Although the baro-receptors normally respond to a raised pulse pressure by increasing their phasic frequency, the tachycardia induced by the direct effect of adrenalin on cardiac muscle is still observed as the stimulus is insufficient to cause a reflex decrease in the heart-rate.

2. Respiratory system

Both sympathetic stimulation (or the administration of noradrenalin) and adrenalin induce dilatation of the bronchi and bronchioles by relaxing the bronchial and bronchiolar muscles. However adrenalin is a more potent bronchodilator than noradrenalin.

3. Gastrointestinal tract

Adrenalin and noradrenalin relax the smooth muscle of the gastrointestinal tract (decreased tone) and inhibit peristalsis; the pyloric and ileocolic sphincters contract.

4. Central nervous system

Adrenalin activates the ascending reticular system (induces arousal). In man it also appears to initiate anxiety, stimulation of breathing, and coarse tremors of the fingers. Noradrenalin appears to be much less potent in producing these effects.

5. Blood

Adrenalin decreases coagulation time (perhaps by increasing the activity of Factor V). It also increases the red blood cell count, the haemoglobin concentration, and the plasma protein concentration. It is believed that these increases are due to simple haemoconcentration due to movement of fluid out of blood into the intercellular spaces. Adrenalin also reduces the eosinophil count, although this effect may be mediated by cortisol from the adrenal cortex (see Chapter 4). Noradrenalin does not appear to produce these various effects on the blood system.

6. Metabolism

a. *Carbohydrate.* Adrenalin is a potent hyperglycaemic agent, due mainly to its actions on the liver and also on the pancreas (see Chapter 8). In the liver it promotes glycogenolysis and gluconeogenesis. Because of the presence in hepatic tissue of a phosphatase which can hydrolyse the glucose 6-phosphate (formed by glycogenolysis) to glucose, the glucose can then diffuse into the blood-stream. Adrenalin also stimulates glycogenolysis in skeletal muscle, but because this tissue does not have the phosphatase, lactic acid is formed from the metabolism of glucose 6-phosphate. The lactic acid reaches the liver where it becomes converted to glucose.

While noradrenalin has little direct effect on carbohydrate metabolism, both the catecholamines can inhibit the glucose-induced secretion of insulin from the β-cells of the islets of Langerhans in the pancreas (see Chapter 8).

b. *Fats.* Both adrenalin and noradrenalin stimulate lipolytic activity in adipose tissue (and muscle), with a resultant increase in the plasma free fatty acid concentration.

c. Adrenalin increases the total oxygen consumption (*calorigenic action*) and increases the basal metabolic rate.

7. The eye

Adrenalin and noradrenalin both dilate the pupil of the eye by stimulating the contraction of the radial smooth muscle.

Metabolism and excretion

Circulating catecholamines are mainly taken up by postsynaptic nerve endings (where they may either be stored in granules or inactivated) and by the liver and kidneys (where they are inactivated). The two principal enzymes involved in the inactivation of the catecholamines are monoamine oxidase (MAO) and catechol-*O*-methyltransferase (COMT). The first of the enzymes (MAO) is located in the mitochondria of the nerve axons, while COMT is present on the postsynaptic cell membranes and in the liver and kidneys. The catecholamines are converted to metadrenalin and normetadrenalin by COMT. Both of these metabolites may be excreted directly in the urine or following conjugation, as glucuronides and sulphates, or following oxidation, via an intermediate aldehyde, to 4-hydroxy-3-methoxymandelic acid (vanillylmandelic acid,

VMA). A somewhat smaller proportion of the intermediate aldehyde is reduced to 4-hydroxy-3-methoxyphenylglycol (HMPG). MAO is responsible for formation of the aldehyde and it may also act directly on the catecholamine, with COMT acting secondarily on the degradation products: 2–3 per cent of the catecholamines are directly excreted in the urine, mostly as conjugates. When large quantities of adrenalin are secreted from the adrenal medulla, for example when a phaeochromocytoma is present, the COMT inactivation mechanism is the more important. This results in a disproportionately high urinary concentration of metadrenalins, although other degradation products, particularly VMA, which is widely used as a diagnostic aid, are present.

CLINICAL DISORDERS OF THE ADRENAL MEDULLA

Tumours of the adrenal medulla

These may, for convenience, be considered in two groups:

1. Neuroblastoma (sympathoblastoma)—ganglioneuroma group

This tumour spectrum ranges from the highly malignant neuroblastoma to the relatively benign ganglioneuroma. Although they commonly produce large amounts of catecholamines, clinical features stemming from this over-production are disproportionately small. They may include changes such as episodic hypertension, sweating attacks, pallor, and diarrhoea, which probably derive from the overproduction of vasoactive intestinal peptide. Extreme catecholamine intoxication is probably avoided by their being metabolized within the tumour before secretion.

2. Phaeochromocytoma

The tumour occurs predominantly in the 25–55 age group and is a rare condition; if it is familial it may be associated with neurofibromatosis (at least 5 per cent) or medullary carcinoma of thyroid. Occasionally phaeo-chromocytoma is one of the abnormalities found in the condition known as multiple endocrine adenomatosis (type II); this is considered in Chapter 9.

The vast majority of phaeochromocytomas (about 85 per cent) occur in the adrenal medulla and are sometimes malignant (5 per cent) and sometimes bilateral (10 per cent). This tumour may also occur anywhere in the sympathetic ganglia of the truncal region; a common site is the organ of Zuckerkandl. Phaeochromocytoma accounts for some 0·1 per cent of all cases of hypertension. However, it is of clinical interest since removal of the tumour results in a restoration of the blood-pressure to normal (claimed to be one of the few totally successful treatments of hypertension); untreated, the prognosis is poor.

CLINICAL FEATURES: Hypertension, which is the cardinal sign, may be intermittent or persistent. The patient may seek advice shortly after the tumour has developed, but the presentation may be delayed for several years. Invariably the patient complains of 'attacks' which may be precipitated by emotion, physical exercise, etc. and which consist of pounding headaches, sweating, pallor, pain in chest or abdomen, apprehension, parasthesiae of the limbs, nausea, and vomiting. If he is observed during an attack the skin is covered with sweat and is usually pale; the pupils are dilated, the limbs feel cold, the blood-pressure is markedly raised, and there may be pyrexia. After an attack there is severe prostration. It is interesting to note that if hypertension persists the condition may be identified by the marked postural hypotension induced by the hypovolaemia.

INVESTIGATIONS: Total urinary metadrenalin output is the most useful single investigation although the somewhat simpler VMA assay is commonly performed. The possible use of radio-enzymatic plasma noradrenalin estimates may in the future be the preferred method of detection. Another test which was and is still used by some is to measure the response to an α-blocking drug. The blood-pressure is measured every 30 seconds for 10 minutes. Interspersed between several intravenous saline injections, one injection of 5 mg of phentolamine is given, the blood-pressure measurements being continued throughout. A positive test is one in which the blood-pressure falls by an arbitrary value (35/25 mm Hg) within a few minutes. Unfortunately the changes when they occur may not be a reliable diagnostic test.

Tests which stimulate the release of adrenalin are dangerous.

TREATMENT: When the tumour has been localized it is removed surgically. An excessive amount of pressor hormones may be released due to surgical manipulation of the gland. It is therefore essential that in the pre-operative period an α-blocker such as phenoxybenzamine be used (20–60 mg/day for several days in divided doses). In addition to the routine pre-operative sedation, tranquillizers such as diazepam should be administered for some 72 hours prior to operation. During the operation any marked elevation of blood-pressure induced by the sudden release of catecholamines can be overcome by the intravenous administration of phentolamine. Careful pre-operative preparation should prevent any severe fall of blood-pressure resulting from the hypovolaemia during the surgical procedure. However it may still be necessary to give blood transfusion (500–1500 ml). If the hypotension persists noradrenalin should be given intravenously in saline.

4 The adrenal cortex

PHYSIOLOGY

The adrenal cortex can be considered as an endocrine gland quite distinct from the adrenal medulla. It is not controlled by direct innervation, but by the action of other hormones and by variations of plasma concentrations of certain chemical substances. It secretes steroid (lipid-soluble) hormones which either control salt and water balance (mineralocorticoids), or regulate general metabolism (glucocorticoids), although their actions are not sharply differentiated. Small and relatively unimportant amounts of sex hormones are also normally secreted by the adrenal cortex. Extirpation of the adrenal cortices is rapidly fatal, so that, unlike the adrenal medullae, they play a vital role in the normal homeostatic regulation of many important metabolic functions.

Anatomy, histology, and development

The adrenal cortex is the outermost part of the adrenal gland, and consists of three relatively distinct layers of cells. The outermost layer is called the zona glomerulosa. This zone is relatively narrow and consists of small cells grouped together in poorly defined clusters. The wider middle zone is called the zona fasciculata and consists of larger cells which are arranged in parallel chains running radially down towards the centre of the gland. The innermost zone, the zona reticularis, consists of cells which are similar to those of the zona fasciculata, but are arranged as an interconnecting network. The arterial blood-supply to the adrenal gland has been described previously (see Chapter 3).

The mineralocorticoids (aldosterone) and glucocorticoids (cortisol)

Synthesis, storage, and release

The hormones of the adrenal cortex are all derived from cholesterol which can itself be synthesized within the gland or taken up from the circulation. The adrenocortical hormones are therefore steroid hormones with a common structure, the cyclopentanoperhydrophenanthrene nucleus. The hormones may conveniently be considered in three groups according to their principal effects: mineralocorticoids, glucocorticoids, and sex hormones. The first two groups of hormones have 21 carbon atoms in their chemical structures (see Fig. 4.1) and are sometimes called C-21 steroids. All C-21 steroids from the adrenal gland have some mineralo- and glucocorticoid activities. The sex hormones from the adrenal cortex are normally synthesized in small quantities relative to the gonadal secretions in the adult. These hormones are mainly

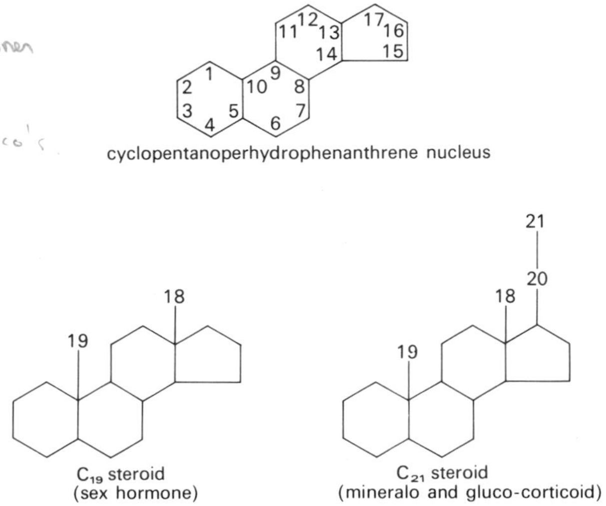

Cortical sex hormones
= C_{19}

Mineralo-gluco's
C_{21}

cyclopentanoperhydrophenanthrene nucleus

C_{19} steroid
(sex hormone)

C_{21} steroid
(mineralo and gluco-corticoid)

Fig.4.1   The basic structures of the steroid hormones.

androgens, containing 19 carbon atoms in their chemical structure, and are therefore sometimes called C-19 steroids.

The main mineralocorticoid in man is aldosterone. This hormone is synthesized from cholesterol which is converted to pregnenolone and then to progesterone. Progesterone is first converted to 11-desoxycorticosterone in the presence of the enzyme 21β-hydroxylase, which is then·converted to corticosterone in the presence of 11β-hydroxylase; this is hydroxylated to 18-hydroxycorticosterone; the enzyme 18-hydroxysteroid dehydrogenase finally converts the 18-hydroxycorticosterone to aldosterone. The enzyme 18-hydroxysteroid dehydrogenase is present only in the zona glomerulosa, and aldosterone can therefore be synthesized only in this part of the adrenal cortex.

Cortisol, which is the principal glucocorticoid in humans, is also synthesized from the progesterone derived from cholesterol. However, progesterone is then converted to 17α-hydroxyprogesterone in the presence of 17α-hydroxylase, an enzyme which is present only in the zonae fasciculata and reticularis. Another enzyme, 21β-hydroxylase is involved in the subsequent conversion of 17α-hydroxyprogesterone to 11-desoxycortisol, which is ultimately converted to cortisol in the presence of 11β-hydroxylase (Fig. 4.2).

Of the androgens secreted by the adrenal cortex, dehydroepiandrosterone (DHEA) is the most important, being secreted in greatest quantities. Significant quantities of these hormones may only be produced if the adrenal cortex is hyperactive in disease, when the effects of excess androgens (and occasionally of oestrogens) may be observed. In this chapter, only the principal mineralocorticoid aldosterone, and the principal glucocorticoid cortisol, will be considered.

Cholesterol, the original precursor molecule for steroid hormone synthesis,

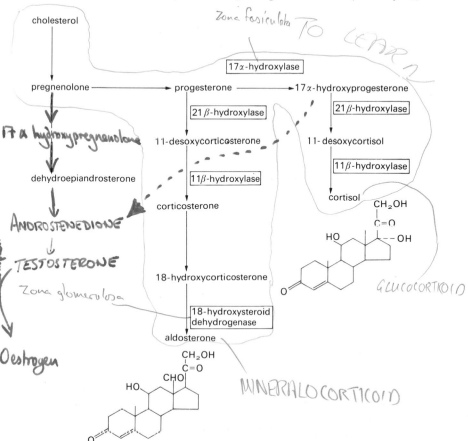

Fig.4.2 The principal metabolites produced in the synthesis pathway of corticosteroids in the adrenal glands, and the chief enzymes involved.

is stored mainly within cytoplasmic lipid droplets in the adrenal cortical cells. The various hormones are stored in only very small quantities. Stimulation of adrenal cells through various control mechanisms therefore induces new synthesis and release of hormone. The secretion rate for aldosterone normally ranges from between 0·1 and 0·4 μmol/24 h whereas cortisol is secreted in far greater quantities, usually varying between 30 and 80 μmol/24 h in humans. Once in the blood approximately 75 per cent of cortisol is tightly but reversibly bound to a plasma glycoprotein called transcortin, which also has a high affinity for other corticosteroids such as desoxycorticosterone and corticosterone. Only about 10 per cent of the cortisol in the blood is in the free and active state, the remainder being loosely bound to plasma albumin. If the total peak concentration (highest normal level) exceeds 850 nmol/l, the free cortisol rises disproportionately because the binding capacity of transcortin is saturated, and albumin binds only a small quantity of the hormone. Aldosterone has a lower affinity than cortisol for transcortin and furthermore, since it is released in much smaller quantities, it does not seriously compete for binding sites on the carrier protein.

Of interest is the observation that in the normal individual the secretion of cortisol follows a diurnal variation which closely follows the diurnal variation of corticotrophin release from the adenohypophysis. The plasma corticotrophin and cortisol levels rise during sleep to reach highest levels in the morning soon after waking up. The levels then decrease to reach lowest values in the evening. This diurnal variation appears to depend on some inherent property of the central nervous system, possibly hypothalamic, which controls corticotrophin release and thus cortisol secretion.

Aldosterone

Actions

The principal effect of aldosterone is to stimulate sodium reabsorption from the distal convoluted tubule; it also acts on sweat glands, gastric glands, and saliva in a similar manner. Sodium reabsorption from the distal convoluted tubule is regulated by a mechanism which involves the exchange of sodium ions in the distal tubular lumen for potassium or hydrogen ions in the extracellular fluid. As a result the control of the extracellular fluid (ECF) volume is influenced by aldosterone, provided that neurohypophysial function is normal. An increased sodium reabsorption raises plasma osmolality, which stimulates the hypothalamic osmo-receptors, resulting in the release of increased quantities of antidiuretic hormone (arginine vasopressin) from the neurohypophysis. Antidiuretic hormone increases the permeability of collecting ducts and thus increases water reabsorption (see Chapter 2). This process continues until plasma osmolality is restored and the stimulus to the osmo-receptors removed. Thus one function of aldosterone is to participate in the control of the extracellular fluid (ECF) volume. When aldosterone is produced in excess, oedema rarely develops because of an 'escape mechanism'. As the ECF volume rises the glomerular filtration rate (GFR) of the kidney increases, this resulting in an increased urine excretion. Generally an expansion of the ECF occurs until the volume has increased by approximately 15 per cent after which the 'escape' phenomenon operates. Whether other mechanisms including a natriuretic hormone operate has not yet been clarified.

Another mineralocorticoid, 11-desoxycorticosterone, has similar effects on sodium reabsorption and potassium excretion, but is much less important physiologically. These hormones thus act to conserve sodium and are of importance in maintaining homeostasis. It must be remembered that while the primary effect of aldosterone and other mineralocorticoids is to increase total body sodium levels, it also has a secondary, but nevertheless important function in controlling the potassium levels in the plasma.

Control of release

The release of aldosterone is controlled by various factors, including a direct effect of plasma sodium and potassium concentrations. Either a 10 per cent decrease in the plasma sodium or a 10 per cent increase in plasma potassium concentration appears to stimulate the synthesis and release of aldosterone. Corticotrophin (ACTH) from the adenohypophysis stimulates the conversion of cholesterol to pregnenolone and can therefore also stimulate aldosterone secretion. However, corticotrophin is not a major factor in the control of aldosterone production, its primary action being the control of cortisol synthesis and release. The possibility that an unidentified substance from the brain called adrenoglomerulotrophin is also involved in regulating aldosterone production has not been totally discounted.

One important control mechanism for the secretion of aldosterone involves the renin-angiotensin system. Renin is an enzyme synthesized and stored in specialized cells located along the terminal part of the afferent arterioles of the renal glomerulus, called juxta-glomerular (JG) cells. These specialized cells constitute part of the juxtaglomerular apparatus (JGA). Following stimulation of the JGA, renin is released into the blood where it acts on a plasma protein called angiotensinogen, synthesized in the liver, to split off a decapeptide called angiotensin I. This molecule is then rapidly converted to an octapeptide, angiotensin II, by a circulating 'converting enzyme'. Angiotensin II stimulates the cells of the zona glomerulosa to produce aldosterone; it is also a potent vasoconstrictor when present in the circulation in large amounts (see Fig. 4.3). It is generally believed that the stimulus for renin release is a decrease in the renal arteriolar blood-pressure which would reduce blood-flow to the kidney. This may result from a generalized fall of systemic blood-pressure either due to a decrease in blood-volume following haemorrhage or salt and water loss, or by abnormally prolonged pooling of the blood in the legs when an upright posture is assumed (postural hypotension). These changes in blood-volume and pressure reduce the frequency of discharge from the baroreceptors in the carotid sinus and aortic arch which results in increased sympathetic activity, inducing generalized arteriolar constriction, including the afferent arteriole to the glomerulus. The specialized cells respond to this change by releasing renin. Alternatively the increased sympathetic activity may result in a direct stimulation of JG cells via adrenergic renal sympathetic nerve fibres.

Cortisol

Actions

The most important naturally occurring glucocorticoids in humans are cortisol and corticosterone, with the derivative cortisone being a potentially active steroid since it can be converted to cortisol in the liver and other tissues. The important physiological effect of glucocorticoids is on carbohydrate metabolism, although this effect is closely associated with actions involving protein and fat metabolism.

Cortisol stimulates hepatic gluconeogenesis which results initially in increased deposition of glycogen in the liver. Gluconeogenesis may be defined as the formation of glucose from non-carbohydrate precursors such as amino acids or glycerol. Any excess glucose synthesized enters the blood-stream and may produce hyperglycaemia; cortisol also antagonizes the peripheral action of insulin on glucose uptake, enhancing the hyperglycaemia. The increased

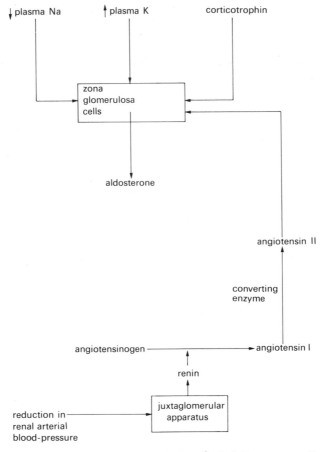

Fig.4.3   The principal factors involved in the control of aldosterone secretion.

gluconeogenesis is principally the result of another important action of cortisol, the stimulation of protein catabolism. This effect can, when the hormone is produced in excess, cause severe wasting of the muscles. In addition cortisol inhibits amino acid uptake and protein synthesis in peripheral tissues (muscle, skin, bone, etc.) while stimulating these effects in the liver. The increased quantities of amino acids in the liver may then be converted to glucose through the gluconeogenic pathway. Cortisol affects fat metabolism, especially when large amounts of hormone are secreted, to produce a centripetal distribution of fat (increased deposition in the facial and truncal areas). The redistribution is associated with an increased lipolysis in adipose tissue, and results in hyperlipidaemia and hypercholesterolaemia. The stretching of the skin over the new fat depots together with loss of its elasticity due to enhanced protein catabolism which can occur when glucocorticoids are secreted in excess result in striae which, as blood seeps into the spaces left by the catabolized collagen, become purple. The glucocorticoids also have some mineralocorticoid activity on salt and water balance, this effect becoming important when the hormones are produced in large quantities.

Other effects of cortisol are observed when the hormone is present in excess. Somatotrophin secretion from the adenohypophysis is decreased. The effect of vitamin D metabolites on the absorption of calcium from the gut is antagonized, while the excretion of calcium by the kidneys is increased. This latter effect is at least partially due to an increased GFR. The various effects on calcium metabolism, together with increased catabolism of bone protein induced by cortisol directly and the impairment of somatotrophin release, probably combine to cause osteoporosis—one of the symptoms of excess glucocorticoid secretion. Another effect is a decrease in the numbers of eosinophils, basophils, and lymphocytes in the blood, whereas the neutrophils as well as the erythrocytes, platelets, and plasma proteins increase.

Large quantities of circulating cortisol also induce certain very important but poorly understood effects which are of considerable clinical value. It inhibits the normal inflammatory process which occurs when tissue is damaged. In the normal process, increased permeability of the capillary walls results in the diffusion of plasma-like fluid into the damaged area together with the migration of leucocytes across the capillary membranes (diapedesis). Lysosomal membranes within the leucocytes rupture, releasing various proteolytic enzymes which then destroy damaged cells and their constituents. Collagen fibres are subsequently formed to repair the original damage. Cortisol blocks all stages of this process thereby preventing the normal repair of damaged tissues, but this action means that the hormone can be used to advantage in certain inflammatory conditions such as rheumatoid arthritis. It may be the stabilizing action of cortisol on lysosomal membranes which is of therapeutic importance. It must not be forgotten however that the healing of wounds may be delayed by inhibiting the formation of collagen fibres.

Another important effect of excess cortisol is its immunosuppressive action. The inhibition of the normal immune response results from the gradual destruction of lymphoid tissue with a resultant decrease in antibody production, as well as a decrease in the numbers of eosinophils, basophils, and lymphocytes. This action is beneficial during transplant and graft operations, although it renders the patient more susceptible to the subversive, uncontrolled spread of an infection throughout the body.

Excess cortisol also has anti-allergic properties, probably due partly to inhibition of the intracellular synthesis of histamine in mast cells and basophils. When an antigen reacts with a tissue antibody on a mast cell, the mast cell ruptures with the subsequent release of histamine which induces capillary dilatation. Capillary membrane permeability is increased, allowing the movement of plasma into the intercellular spaces. The resultant decrease in venous eturn lowers the blood-pressure, this being one of the features of anaphylactic shock. In man the fall of blood-pressure is enhanced because of the additional arteriolar dilatation. In addition histamine causes some smooth muscle contraction, in particular that of bronchioles. It also stimulates salivary, pancreatic, gastric, and intestinal secretions. Thus cortisol (which inhibits histamine synthesis and release) alleviates some of the allergic responses. Part of the anti-allergic action of excess cortisol may be due to other effects such as the inhibition of kinin synthesis, the decreased production of antibodies and the stabilization of lysosomal membranes.

Major stresses such as severe trauma, pyrogens, injections of histamine, acute hypoglycaemia, and emotional stimuli all induce a rapid increase in corticotrophin secretion from the adenohypophysis and a consequent increase in cortisol secretion, and it has been suggested that these hormones may play some role in combating the harmful effects of stressful situations. However, it must not be assumed that increased quantities of cortisol are necessarily beneficial to the organisms's response to stress.

Control of release

It has been known for some time that hypophysectomy results in a gradual atrophy of the two innermost zones of the adrenal cortex—the zona fasciculata and the zona reticularis, and it is now well established that the synthesis and secretion of the glucocorticoids and the adrenal sex steroids, are under the control of the adenohypophysial hormone corticotrophin. The diurnal variation in the secretory pattern of cortisol is directly related to the diurnal variation of corticotrophin release, as mentioned earlier in the chapter. The stimulatory effect of corticotrophin is believed to be mediated by the activation of adenyl cyclase through a membrane-bound receptor, with a subsequent increase in cyclic AMP concentrations. Cyclic AMP may then stimulate the conversion of cholesterol to pregnenolone, and the various conversions of pregnenolone to progesterone and ultimately to cortisol, by activating the various enzyme systems involved (see Chapter 10). The release of the adenohypophysial hormone corticotrophin is itself controlled mainly from the hypothalamus through the mediation of the corticotrophin-releasing factor (CRF). The negative feedback system involving cortisol and other glucocorticoids has been identified at both hypothalamic and adenohypophysial levels (see Fig. 4.4), as discussed in Chapter 1.

CLINICAL DISORDERS

The introduction of radioimmune assays has considerably advanced our understanding of disorders of this gland and provided us with an important diagnostic tool. However, these assays have at the same time created new problems by establishing the existence of 'borderline' patients in whom it is difficult to distinguish whether or not there is an adrenal disorder. The basic disturbances of adrenocortical hormones are discussed in this chapter.

Individual hormone disorders

Aldosterone

Excess

Hyperaldosteronism is caused by a sustained high secretion of aldosterone from one or both adrenal cortices, and can be divided into two categories.

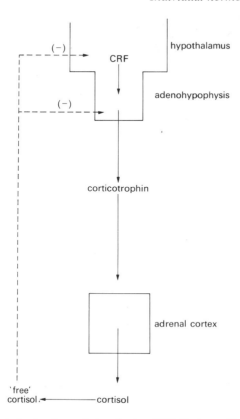

Fig.4.4   The control system for cortisol production. CRF: Corticotrophin releasing factor.

a. Primary aldosteronism: in this condition there is an autonomous secretion of excess aldosterone by the adrenal cortex (unilateral or bilateral), without involvement of the renin–angiotensin system.
b. Secondary aldosteronism: high aldosterone secretion is induced by the enhanced levels of angiotensin II due to a high plasma renin activity (PRA) which may result from a variety of causes.

The effects produced in primary and secondary states are often very different. In primary aldosteronism the clinical picture can be derived from an understanding of the physiological actions of aldosterone, while in the secondary variety the numerous and varied causes of the raised renin usually dominate the clinical picture. In both conditions the aldosterone level is raised, but the important biochemical difference is that in primary aldosteronism the angiotensin levels are depressed whereas in secondary aldosteronism they are elevated.

Primary aldosteronism (Conn's syndrome)

This is due in the majority of cases to single or multiple adrenal adenomata which are usually unilateral but may occasionally be bilateral; the tumour is very rarely malignant. Of the remainder the disorder is usually of unknown aetiology, and arises from a hyperplasia of the zona glomerulosa.

CLINICAL FEATURES: These patients usually have hypertension due to salt and water retention. However, there are often no secondary effects from the hypertension, and retinopathy and cardiomegaly if present are usually mild; peripheral oedema is rare in the absence of cardiac failure. Hypokalaemia gives rise to other symptoms such as parasthesiae, muscle weakness, and polyuria, although these occur only if the serum potassium level falls below 3·0 mmol/l at which concentration electrocardiographic changes may be seen: ST depression, flattening of T waves, and the appearance of U waves. Frequently glycosuria is detected. Only on rare occasions are symptoms referrable to local involvement by the adrenal tumour.

INVESTIGATIONS:

1. Plasma potassium and other electrolytes are routinely estimated. The diagnosis must be considered likely if there is hypokalaemia in a patient with asymptomatic hypertension, provided other causes of hypokalaemia such as vomiting, diarrhoea, and diuretic therapy are excluded. Further evidence is an inappropriately high daily urinary potassium excretion in the presence of low plasma potassium levels. Normokalaemic primary aldosteronism is uncommon. Other electrolyte abnormalities sometimes present, including hypernatraemia and hypochloraemic alkalosis. Cushing's syndrome must be excluded as it may also present with hypokalaemia and hypertension.

2. The diagnosis is established by the finding of high plasma aldosterone and low plasma angiotensin II (measured as plasma renin–angiotensin, PRA) levels provided these are measured under standard conditions, as both are altered by dietary sodium and protein intake, and by posture.

3. After establishing the diagnosis an attempt may be made to obtain adrenal vein samples in order to determine whether the excess aldosterone is unilateral or bilateral in origin.

4. These tumours are usually avascular and arteriography is usually of little value.

TREATMENT: The treatment of choice is the surgical removal of single or multiple adenomata. This usually results in a rapid fall in blood-pressure and the plasma levels of electrolytes revert to normal. If an adenoma has not been demonstrated pre-operatively, the adrenal is explored at operation, and if none are found, provided the diagnosis has been established, the whole of one and one-half of the other adrenal is removed. Medical treatment with an aldosterone antagonist, spironolactone (50 mg 8-hourly or more) can be given pre-operatively with good results. In patients who are unsuitable for surgery this drug therapy can be used often with highly satisfactory results despite occasional adverse effects which include gynaecomastia, impotence, and lassitude.

Secondary aldosteronism

A rise in circulating angiotensin II levels due to increased renin release stimulates the adrenal cortex to produce and release increased quantities of aldosterone. This physiological reflex is designed to conserve sodium under conditions of physical stress, such as haemorrhage or salt and water depletion (e.g. diarrhoea and vomiting). In disease this physiological mechanism may become deranged; the volume receptors are believed to operate inappropriately in the nephrotic syndrome, cardiac failure, and in cirrhosis of the liver with ascites. Hence in these conditions aldosterone secretion increases despite the raised extracellular volume. Furthermore, should the blood-supply to the juxtaglomerular apparatus be impaired as in accelerated (malignant) hypertension or renal artery stenosis, there is enhanced secretion of aldosterone. However, the commonest cause of secondary aldosteronism is now diuretic therapy. The causes of secondary aldosteronism are given in Table 4.1.

In hypertensive patients the distinction between primary aldosteronism (adrenal tumour, or benign hyperplasia) and secondary aldosteronism is made by measuring the PRA, thereby estimating the concentration of angiotensin. Secondary aldosteronism and hypokalaemia may occur with or without hypertension, and Table 4.2 summarizes the conditions in which this may occur. Detailed discussion of secondary aldosteronism is outside the scope of this book.

Deficiency

Adrenocortical insufficiency may also be conveniently divided into two main categories: primary insufficiency due to disease of the adrenal gland itself

Table 4.1.   Causes of secondary aldosteronism

1. Poor renal perfusion:

   a. loss of effective blood volume:
     i.   dehydration
     ii. haemorrhage
     iii. loss of sodium and water into extravascular space:
        1. cardiac failure and oedema
        2. cirrhosis and ascites
        3. nephrotic syndrome
     iv. salt-loosing nephritis

   b. mechanical obstruction of renal artery or arterioles:
     i.   accelerated hypertension/fibrinoid necrosis
     ii. fibromuscular hyperplasia
     iii. atheroma
     iv. renal arteriolar damage or distortion

2. Primary excess of renin. There are two rare conditions:
     i.   Hyperplasia of the juxtaglomerular apparatus (Bartter's syndrome)
     ii. Renin-secreting renal tumours.

3. The commonest cause of secondary aldosteronism is now diuretic therapy.

Table 4.2   Secondary aldosteronism and hypokalaemia, with or without hypertension

Without hypertension	With hypertension
Diuretic therapy	Diuretic therapy
Low sodium diet	Accelerated hypertension
Nephrotic syndrome	Renovascular hypertension
Cirrhosis	Oral contraceptive hypertension
Cardiac failure	Juxtaglomerular cell tumour†
‡Bartter's syndrome	High liquorice intake

† Juxtaglomerular cell tumours results in excess renin secretion. This is a rare syndrome.
‡ Bartter's syndrome is secondary aldosteronism characterized by juxtaglomerular cell hyperplasia, high renin and aldosterone levels, and an inability to thrive.

(Addison's disease), and secondary insufficiency consequent upon absent or low levels of corticotrophin. The latter cause of adrenal atrophy results from either disease of the adenohypophysis or the suppression of the hypothalamic–adenohypophysial system during the administration of high doses of exogenous steroids and which may continue for a period after withdrawal of the steroid.

One important difference between primary and secondary states is that in the former there is a decrease in mineralocorticoid (aldosterone) and glucocorticoid (cortisol) hormone concentrations whereas in the latter aldosterone levels are near-normal. Adrenal insufficiency may present either as a catastrophic acute emergency or as a chronic disorder. Some diseases of the adrenal cortex are usually associated with an acute onset of adrenal failure. However, it must be emphasized that those conditions which usually have an insidious onset may, if an infection or stress is superimposed, present as an acute adrenal failure. The causes of primary adrenal insufficiency are given in Table 4.3.

Table 4.3   Causes of primary adrenal insufficiency

1. Chronic primary adrenal insufficiency (Addison's disease):
   a. autoimmune adrenalitis is the commonest cause and is associated with serum adrenal antibodies, and other autoimmune diseases such as pernicious anaemia and thyroiditis
   b. tuberculosis of the adrenal gland
   c. rarer causes include infiltration of the glands with metastatic carcinoma or amyloid, fungal infection, or haemochromatosis

2. Acute primary adrenal insufficiency:
   a. any case of chronic primary adrenal insufficiency when stressed by infection or operation
   b. septicaemia with adrenal haemorrhage (Waterhouse-Friderichsen syndrome); usually caused by meningococcal septicaemia
   c. following bilateral adrenalectomy without replacement therapy
   d. adrenal haemorrhage occurs rarely either with anti-coagulant overdose or with a breech delivery at birth

Primary adrenal insufficiency

CLINICAL FEATURES: In the acute state the usual features are vomiting, abdominal pain, extreme muscular weakness, dehydration leading to hypotension, confusion, and even coma. This condition (Addisonian crisis) is fortunately rare (Chapter 11). The chronic condition has an insidious onset and the initial symptoms, which are usually non-specific, consist of tiredness, weakness, anorexia, vague abdominal pains, vomiting, weight loss, and dizzy spells. A more specific sign (and sometimes complaint) is increased pigmentation, especially of the exposed areas of the body, points of friction or pressure, creases of the palms, freckles (i.e. parts normally pigmented), buccal mucosa, the nipples, the genitalia, and scars. It is important to realize that the pigmentation may not be brown; it may be blue or grey. It is claimed that pigmentation of the mouth is characteristic of Addison's disease, provided there is no coloured ancestry. In some patients areas of depigmentation (vitiligo) may occur in the pigmented area and occasionally pigmentation is absent (Plate 4.1). The decreased blood-pressure is due to the sodium loss and fluid depletion induced by the aldosterone deficiency, and also to the 'poor vascular tone' which is claimed to result from the low plasma cortisol level. Hypotension may only be postural dizzy episodes occurring when the upright position is assumed. Hypoglycaemic phases (confusion, bizarre behaviour, etc. (Chapter 8), but rarely coma) may occur in the early morning or if a meal is omitted. These symptoms and signs are common and non-specific, and in the absence of characteristic pigmentation the diagnosis of Addison's disease may not be made.

The underlying cause of the disease may give rise to special clinical findings such as haemoptysis and focal lung signs in pulmonary tuberculosis or bronchial carcinoma (see Table 4.3).

INVESTIGATIONS:

1. Simple investigations such as measurement of plasma urea and electrolytes are performed. A low plasma sodium concentration with high blood urea and potassium levels are suggestive of Addison's disease. Repeated plasma cortisol estimations throughout the day and the 24-h estimation of urinary free cortisol are of value. Low levels of plasma cortisol and urinary free cortisol are evidence in favour of Addison's disease.

2. The criterion for the diagnosis of Addison's disease is the demonstration of an impaired output of cortisol with a high circulating plasma corticotrophin level. Impaired cortisol output may become apparent only on stimulation with exogenous corticotrophin (Synacthen test), since basal cortisol levels can be maintained in the normal range by maximal stimulation of the adrenal cortex with high levels of endogenous corticotrophin; nevertheless, cortisol levels are usually low. The failure of the low basal plasma cortisol to rise significantly after the administration of Synacthen is regarded as a reliable test.

3. The plasma corticotrophin level distinguishes primary from secondary adrenal atrophy, with high levels occurring in the primary disorder. The low levels of the hormone in secondary adrenal atrophy due to

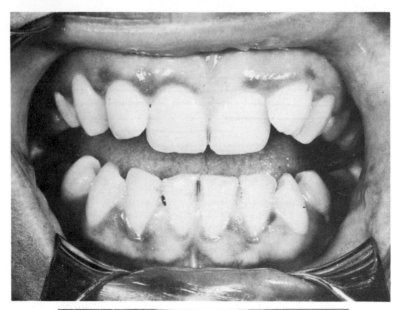

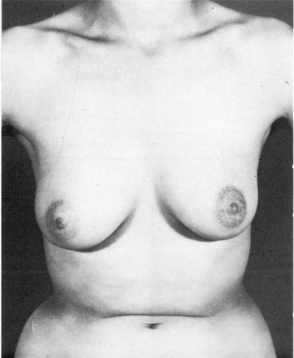

Plate 4.1 The characteristic pigmentation of the gum margins (a), and of both sides of the waist area (b). This patient wore a garment which constricted the waist.

adenohypophysial disease are poorly defined from normal values, as the majority of assay techniques are insufficiently sensitive.

4. Adrenal antibodies should be sought to confirm autoimmune adrenalitis, as this is the commonest cause of Addison's disease.

5. Radiography of the chest may reveal pulmonary tuberculosis, or bronchial carcinoma.

Abdominal radiography may show adrenal calcification in tuberculous adrenal disease.

TREATMENT: The treatment of the acute crisis is considered in Chapter 11, where it is emphasized that treatment precedes confirmatory laboratory results. In the chronic non-critical case investigations may precede treatment. Full replacement requires 20–30 mg cortisol in 24 h in two or three divided doses in the adult, but frequently this has to be supplemented with fludro-cortisone (a mineralocorticoid) 0·05–0·1 mg/day. It is of particular impor-tance to ensure that children are not given an excessive dose of cortisol as this will impair growth. These patients cannot increase the output of adrenal hormones during stress and are therefore at risk in stressful situations such as infection, operation, or trauma. It is essential for them to carry a card giving details of their disease and their dose of corticosteroids, in addition to a vial of steroids. These patients should be routinely reviewed in order to ensure that replacement therapy is adequate, and to continually exclude any underlying disease such as pulmonary tuberculosis. The patients should be instructed to increase their dosage of glucocorticoids if they develop an infection, injury, etc. For an upper respiratory infection a temporary increase of double the dose of cortisol is usually sufficient. In stressful situations such as routine labour or simple surgical procedures, 100 mg of hydrocortisone are given parenterally at operation or at the start of labour. If there are no complications 100 mg are given either intramuscularly or orally every 6 h for 24 h thereafter. Sub-sequently the dose of the hormone, is now only given by mouth, is decreased by 50 per cent every day until the maintenance dose is achieved. In major operations 100 mg of hydrocortisone are given parenterally every 4 h during the operation and during the 48–72 h postoperative period. Thereafter, the dose is reduced at the same rate as described previously. Commonly these patients are unable to eat following major surgery and it is wise to give 1–2 l of saline intravenously every day until the diet is deemed to be adequate.

Secondary adrenal insufficiency

Adenohypophysial disorders have been discussed in Chapter 2. However, another cause of secondary adrenal insufficiency, namely corticosteroid therapy, is now briefly considered.

The dose of cortisol may be such that partial suppression of the adenohy-pophysis is induced such that at times of stress, such as infection and surgical procedures, the secretion of corticotrophin fails to rise sufficiently to produce the required extra cortisol. Sudden withdrawal of steroids after a long period of administration can result in acute adrenal insufficiency. Therefore patients on corticosteroid therapy (sufficient to suppress corticotrophin secretion) must have the quantity gradually reduced over a period of about several months, this being accepted as sufficient time to allow corticotrophin levels to rise and for the output of adrenal cortical hormones to reach normal levels. It is essential to assess the functional capacity of the adrenal cortex before stopping hormone therapy.

Cortisol

Excess (Cushing's syndrome)

Cushing's syndrome is a rare disease predominantly affecting women in the age group 30–50 years. This syndrome is produced by excessive quantities of glucocorticoids, whether these are secreted by the adrenal cortex (endogenous) or administered (exogenous, iatrogenic). Excessive secretion of cortisol may be caused by increased corticotrophin production by the adenohypophysis (Cushing's disease) or ectopic corticotrophin production by a tumour (see Chapter 9), both of which give rise to adrenal hyperplasia. It may also be caused by an independent hypersecretion of cortisol by the adrenal gland due to an adenoma or carcinoma. The commonest cause of the syndrome is oversecretion of adenohypophysial corticotrophin. Often in adenohypophysial corticotrophin hypersecretion, no structural change is found in the pars distalis, but in a small percentage of cases an adenoma is present. Adrenal adenomas are the commonest cause of corticotrophin-independent hypersecretion of cortisol; carcinoma of the adrenal is a rare cause in adults, but has a higher incidence in children. Many of the clinical features of Cushing's syndrome can be predicted by the physiological effects of the hormones secreted.

CLINICAL FEATURES: The clinical picture of Cushing's syndrome can range from the florid, easily recognizable picture to the patient with few signs or symptoms. Some of the more common complaints are proximal muscle weakness with characteristic difficulty in getting out of chairs or climbing stairs, back pain, gain of weight, acne, and in women hairiness and amenorrhoea. There may be a history of recent psychiatric disorder. The obesity is predominantly truncal and there is often a pad of fat between the shoulders ('buffalo hump') (see Plate 4.2). There may be marked wasting of proximal muscles resulting in thin arms and legs which gives rise to the 'lemon on matchsticks' appearance. When present the characteristic red 'moon face' is a striking feature, as are the 'classic' purple striae which are found on the lower abdomen and upper thighs (see Plate 4.3) and these provide clinical evidence in favour of Cushing's syndrome. In addition, the skin is thin and bruises easily. Hirsutism when present may be due to either excess cortisol which induces growth of fine hair, or to the commonly associated excess of androgens which promote the growth of coarse hair (see Plate 4.4). There may be some degree of virilism, which is most marked in patients with carcinoma of the adrenal. On routine examination the majority of patients will be found to have hypertension and, on occasions, glycosuria. On the rare occasions when this syndrome occurs in children, there is stunting of growth.

The classical features of the syndrome are the results of the physiological effects of excess cortisol. Cortisol causes obesity by stimulating the appetite and increasing fat synthesis. It promotes protein catabolism which causes muscle wasting and weakness, and loss of protein in supportive tissues results

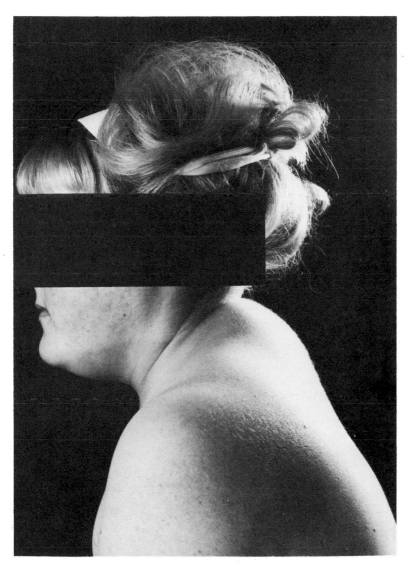

Plate 4.2   This photograph illustrates the typical buffalo hump.

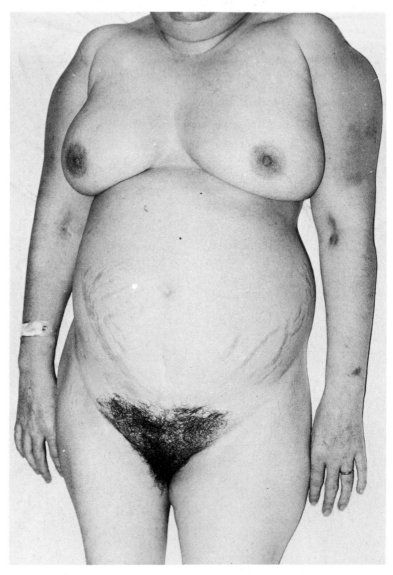

Plate 4.3   This photograph illustrates the truncal obesity and the abdominal striae. Striae can also be observed on the upper outer aspects of the thighs.

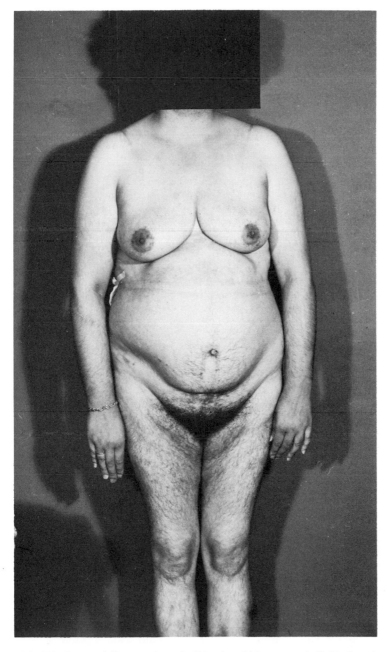

Plate 4.4   This photograph illustrates the marked hirsutism which may occur in Cushing's syndrome.

in striae and bruising, loss of protein bone matrix leads to osteoporosis, vertebral collapse, and even spinal cord compression. A complication of the hypercalcuria probably consequent upon the osteoporosis is renal calculi. Cortisol has some mineralocorticoid activity and in this syndrome causes sodium retention and potassium loss. The hypokalaemia may induce parasthesiae and also contribute to muscle weakness. Sodium retention is accompanied by water retention and is a factor in the development of hypertension. The anti-insulin effects of cortisol impair glucose tolerance, and usually give rise to asymptomatic glycosuria. In addition, the hormone suppresses the inflammatory response and reduces immune defences sometimes making these patients prone to unusual and not easily recognized infections (cryptic infections).

In ectopic corticotrophin production the syndrome is much more acute, often with severe muscle weakness, loss of weight, oedema, and pigmentation. Hypokalaemia is usually profound and there may be electrocardiographic changes (ST depression and U waves), and even loss of renal concentrating ability with polyuria and polydipsia. The underlying carcinoma may give rise to symptoms or signs relative to the organ involved.

INVESTIGATIONS: Investigation is primarily to substantiate the presence of excess circulating cortisol and secondarily to establish the cause:

1. Loss of diurnal rhythm of cortisol secretion is one of the earliest changes, and an elevated level at midnight may indicate the possibility of this disorder. Daily urinary excretion of free cortisol most accurately reflects total cortisol production.

   The excretion of 17-oxogenic and 17-oxosteroids (derived from androgens) are sometimes elevated, the latter increase being common in carcinoma of the adrenal. However, such measurements are not now used to confirm cortisol overproduction.

2. Stress and obesity may both induce high cortisol levels, and difficulty can be experienced in distinguishing clinically between these conditions and Cushing's syndrome. In stress and simple obesity the negative feedback control mechanism between cortisol and corticotrophin is normal. With this information it is now possible to consider the suppression tests which can be used not only to establish the diagnosis, but also to differentiate between adrenal and adenohypophysial causes, and the ectopic secretion of corticotrophin.

   Dexamethasone is used at two dose levels, 0·5 mg (low dosage) or 2 mg (high dosage), either dose of which is given at 6-hourly intervals for 48 h. In stress and simple obesity the response is the same as the normal state in that the low dose of dexamethasone suppresses the secretion of corticotrophin, and produces a decrease of plasma cortisol and urinary free cortisol concentrations. In patients with Cushing's syndrome due to an autonomous adrenal disorder, there is no suppression of cortisol, but if there is hypersecretion of corticotrophin from the adenohypophysis, there may be some fall in cortisol secretion but not as great as in the normal.

   The high dose of dexamethasone usually suppresses the levels of the trophic hormone in Cushing's disease (and correspondingly reduces the cortisol levels), but if there is no reduction either the adrenal gland is the source of the disorder, or the corticotrophin is of ectopic origin.

3. Metyrapone interferes with the hydroxylation of 11-desoxycortisol, causing a fall in the plasma cortisol levels. Administration of this drug in Cushing's disease results in a consequent elevation of corticotrophin and an increased excretion of cortisol precursors. If the disorder is a primary adrenal disease, as in adenoma or carcinoma or a source of ectopic corticotrophin, there is no increase of these metabolites.

4. The corticotrophin level can now be determined in the plasma, and this measurement provides the best and most direct method of distinguishing adrenal from adenohypophysial disorders. While patients with adenohypophysial hypersecretion of corticotrophin have a high plasma level of this hormone, the highest values are found in ectopic secretion; conversely corticotrophin levels are low in patients with adrenal tumours.

5. Radiography of the abdomen may reveal calcification if there is an adrenal tumour. This may displace the kidney which is observed on intravenous pyelography. In Cushing's disease radiography of the skull may reveal enlargement of the sella turcica and erosion of the clinoid processes. Tomography of the fossa may be of value if the routine skull X-ray shows little change. Computerized axial tomography (EMI scan) is not usually of value if the tumour is intrasellar. If the fault is of adrenal origin arteriography of this gland may be considered. In ectopic production of corticotrophin a chest X-ray may reveal a tumour.

6. Examination of the visual field may indicate bitemporal hemianopia if the adenohypophysial tumour is compressing the optic chiasma. However, this is very rare. Minor defects may be detected in less severe cases.

TREATMENT: The urgency of the treatment should be regarded as proportional to the severity of the changes observed. The florid case is regarded as requiring therapy as soon as possible. The treatment is either ablation of the adenohypophysis or bilateral adrenalectomy. Destruction or removal of the adenohypophysis is the procedure adopted for those patients with excess corticotrophin. Hypophysial irradiation has given good results in about 50 per cent of patients. This is usually achieved by the external application of some 4500 rad (45 Gy) or by radioactive implants of yttrium or gold; recently external proton bombardment has met with some success. It must be recalled that this therapy does not induce a remission of the disease for several months and may subsequently give rise to panhypopituitarism. Hypophysial surgery is reserved for those patients with suprasellar extension of the tumour and compression of the optic chiasma. This therapy invariably results in adenohypophysial deficiency and hormone replacement therapy is then required (Chapter 2). Previously bilateral adrenalectomy was advocated for the patient with high levels of corticotrophin, but it is claimed that after the operation the adenohypophysial tumour may grow at an accelerated rate and the patient may develop pigmentation induced by the high level of corticotrophin (Nelson's syndrome). Recently it has been suggested that radiation of the hypophysis followed by bilateral adrenalectomy is the treatment of choice. However, this procedure necessitates not only the replacement of adrenal cortical hormones, but may also occasionally require treatment of any resulting adenohypophysial deficiency. There is, in addition, the operational risk of an adrenalectomy.

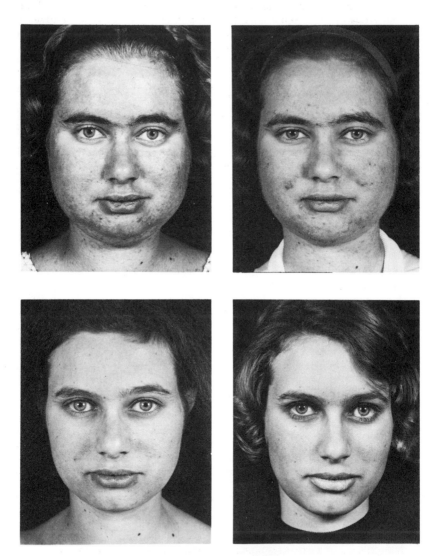

Plate 4.5   This sequence of photographs illustrates a patient with Cushing's syndrome before and after bilateral adrenalectomy. The striking physical changes occur with unexpected rapidity. (a) 11 days before operation; (b) one month after operation; (c) three months after operation; (d) sixteen months after operation.

Tumours of the adrenal should be treated by surgical removal. Both adrenals should be exposed and if a tumour is found in one gland only a unilateral adrenalectomy need be performed. If no tumour is located, bilateral adrenalectomy is carried out because of the likelihood of microadenomata. With adrenal surgery, immediate steroid therapy is given. Subsequently, the dose is reduced to the standard maximum quantity of 20–30 mg of cortisol per 24 h. Even if only one adrenal is removed steroid therapy should be administered as the negative feedback by cortisol on the hypothalamo-adenohypophysial axis may initially be suppressed, but after a few months the hormone is gradually withdrawn. It must be emphasized that patients on a maintenance dose of steroid be warned about the necessity of increasing the dose of the hormone during any infection or stress (see p. 50). It is essential that these patients always possess a card stating that they are on steroid therapy, giving the daily quantity; special bracelets with these details are of value. The photographs show the result of bilateral adrenalectomy and the subsequent improvement in a patient (Plate 4.5).

Carcinoma of the adrenal is often diagnosed after metastases have occurred. If the metastatic deposits synthesize cortisol, postoperative care is difficult. Under these circumstances it is necessary to block the synthesis of this hormone with drugs such as metyrapone (500–750 mg 6-hourly) or aminoglutethimide (250 mg three times daily) together with the administration of sufficient cortisol to meet the requirements of the patient.

In patients who for any reason cannot undergo operation or in patients with ectopic secretion of corticotrophin, metyrapone may also be used with some success. The basic treatment of ectopic secretion is removal, if possible, of the malignant tumour or carcinoid of the lung (Chapter 9). Some patients may survive with the malignant condition and only deteriorate very slowly; in these patients it has been suggested that bilateral adrenalectomy may be worthwhile.

Disorders of hormone synthesis

Clinical disorders may arise due to congenital enzyme defects which impair the synthesis of cortisol and aldosterone. In these circumstances, excess quantities of androgens may be produced. In addition, depending on the site of action of the enzyme involved, there may be an excessive secretion of mineralocorticoids other than aldosterone. However these steroids do not suppress the hypothalamo-adenohypophysial system and the plasma levels of corticotrophin are raised. The excessive release of trophic hormone not only stimulates adrenal cortical secretion but also induces hyperplasia of this gland. As there is adrenal enlargement, this syndrome is usually referred to as congenital adrenal hyperplasia.

The clinical features are dependent upon the severity of the particular enzyme defect, which may be so mild that in order to establish the biochemical diagnosis stimulation with exogenous corticotrophin may be necessary. Little is known of the aetiologies, apart from the fact that they are recessive traits and the conditions may occur in families. Figure 4.5 summarizes the two most common enzyme defects, which are discussed in the following section.

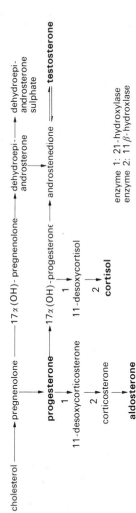

Fig. 4.5   The normal metabolic pathways involved in the synthesis of adrenocortical hormones. Only the site of action of two of the enzymes are indicated because these are the most commonly absent in the rare condition of congenital adrenal hyperplasia. Substances in bold type are the hormones of the adrenal cortex.

1. 21-Hydroxylase deficiency

This is the most frequent defect and yet has an incidence of only approximately 0·01 per cent in patients with adrenal insufficiency. In the absence of this enzyme, 17-hydroxyprogesterone and progesterone are not converted to 11-desoxycortisol (precursor of cortisol) and 11-desoxycorticosterone (precursor of aldosterone) respectively (see Fig. 4.5). The excess of substrate available thus allows an enhanced synthesis and secretion of androgens in response to increased corticotrophin drive. Naturally if the defect is absolute the infant does not survive, because of acute adrenal cortical failure. If the defect is severe, survival is only possible for a short period of time without treatment.

CLINICAL FEATURES: A noticeable feature in both sexes with the less severe defect is early muscular development and advanced bone age. The young boy presents with pseudo-precocious puberty (Chapter 5). Greater interest has focused on the female since the defect when it occurs *in utero* induces masculinization. There may be fusion of the labia to give an apparent scrotum together with hypertrophy of the clitoris. Thus the female may be wrongly registered as a male with hypospadias. If the defect occurs later, there is virilism, in which condition the following changes occur: hirsutism, clitoral enlargement, a coarsening of the voice, recession of the hair line of the forehead, acne, and muscle hypertrophy (Plate 4.6). Not all of these are necessarily present.

INVESTIGATIONS:

1. A buccal smear for Barr bodies or karyotype determination should be carried out in the infant or child in whom there is some difficulty in determining the sex.
2. A raised level of 17-hydroxyprogesterone in the plasma which falls to normal with cortisol therapy is diagnostic of this disorder.
3. Urinary pregnenetriol levels are markedly elevated.
4. In the very mild disorder the plasma levels of cortisol and aldosterone are usually within normal limits.

TREATMENT: The treatment consists of glucocorticoid therapy which both maintains plasma levels of the adrenal hormones and suppresses corticotrophin secretion, thus preventing excess adrenal androgen production. The glucocorticoid of choice is dexamethasone given in divided quantities, but the dose at night is 50 per cent of the daily dose and is given as close to midnight as possible. This technique suppresses the overnight release of corticotrophin. In children it is technically difficult to adjust the dose of dexamethasone because the smallest tablet is 1 mg. It is preferable to use cortisol thrice daily in these circumstances, but again the largest dose is given at night. Initially, higher doses may be needed to depress the pregnenetriol levels. If there is a marked salt loss, a mineralocorticoid is required such as fludrocortisone (0·1 mg daily).

2. 11β-Hydroxylase deficiency

In this condition cortisol and aldosterone synthesis are both decreased. The

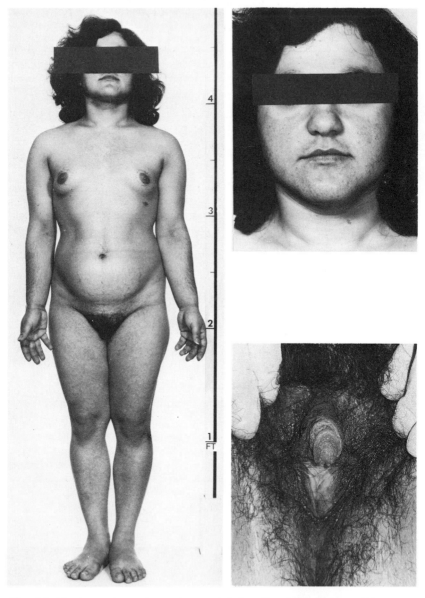

Plate 4.6   The changes that may be seen in congenital adrenal hyperplasia. The truncal hirsutism is not readily seen, but the facial hirsutism and acne are apparent. The clitoral changes are striking. The disorder was due to a 21-hydroxylase deficiency.

resulting high level of corticotrophin stimulates the available metabolic pathways resulting in excess androgen production. Mineralocorticoid activity results from the enhanced secretion of 11-desoxycortisol and 11-desoxycorticosterone (see Fig. 4.5).

CLINICAL FEATURES: The clinical picture is again one of virilism. hypertension is induced by, it is claimed, the excess of 11-desoxycortisol and 11-desoxycorticosterone.

INVESTIGATIONS:

1. Excessive quantities of 17-oxosteroid are excreted in the urine in this condition. This excretion decreases to normal levels following the administration of steroid hormone.

2. If it is possible to measure 11-desoxycortisol in the plasma, raised levels will be detected.

3. 11-oxygenation index (11-OI). This index reflects the efficiency of the last stages of cortisol biosynthesis. It measures the ratio of adrenocortical steroids without oxygenation at C-11 position to those with oxygenation at C-11. It is carried out on a random sample of urine (20 ml) from infants of more than 8 days old, when maturation of the cortisol biosynthesis pathway has occurred. The upper limit of normal is 0·7, and values of 0·9–6·7 have been observed in congenital adrenal hypertrophy.

TREATMENT: The treatment is glucocorticoid given in sufficient quantities to suppress 17-oxosteroid excretion to normal.

5. The gonads

PHYSIOLOGY

Each half of this chapter has, by necessity, been considered in two parts, the first being concerned with the male gonads (the testes) and the second with the female gonads (the ovaries) including such relevant topics as pregnancy, the feto-placental unit, parturition, and lactation. Since genetic sex differentiation and early embryonic gonadal development are two topics which are fundamental and closely related to the testes and the ovaries, these are considered first.

Anatomy and development

The human somatic cell contains 46 chromosomes in pairs, 22 pairs being somatic (autosomal), and the twenty-third being the sex-determinant chromosomes. The female sex is genetically determined by a pair of X-chromosomes, while the male has one X-chromosome and one Y-chromosome. Cell division of a parent germ cell by meiosis (first and second meiotic divisions), which takes place in the gonads, results ultimately in the separation of the chromosomes in each pair so that the daughter cells formed each have half the total number of chromosomes (i.e. 23 chromosomes). Propagation of the species therefore depends on the fusion of two daughter cells each with half the number of chromosomes (haploid) to form a new cell with the full complement of 46 chromosomes (diploid). One daughter cell comes from the mother and the other from the father. The formation of daughter cells (gametes) by meiosis is called gametogenesis. The new cell with the XX sex chromosomes develops into a genetic female, while the cell with the XY-chromosomes develops into the genetic male, the Y-chromosome being ultimately the genetic sex determinant (see Fig. 5.1).

In the embryo primordial germ cells migrate from the yolk sac to the genital ridge of mesoderm on the dorsal wall of the developing abdominal cavity. Proliferation of the cells of the genital ridge, incorporating the primordial germ cells, results in the development of the primitive gonads beside the mesonephros. These primitive gonads are initially identical in both sexes. Up to the sixth week of intrauterine life both Mullerian (female) and Wolffian (male) primitive genital tract systems develop and it is only after the sixth week that the gonads begin to differentiate into testes or ovaries.

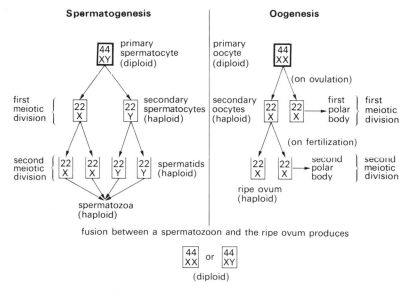

Fig.5.1   The production of spermatozoa (spermatogenesis) and a ripe ovum (oogenesis).

The testes (androgens)

Anatomy, histology, and development

From the sixth week of intrauterine life the primitive testes suppress the further development of the female Mullerian system possibly by secreting an unidentified 'Mullerian regression factor'. Sex cords which contain the germ cells develop from the coelomic epithelium covering the genital ridge to become the seminiferous tubules. The development of interstitial cells from the surrounding mesoderm results in the production of androgens (male sex steroids) primarily testosterone, which then stimulate the formation of the vas deferens from the Wolffian duct. Should failure of primitive testicular function occur and the Mullerian duct system remain, an outwardly normal but incomplete female genital tract system develops in a male genotype. In the seventh to eighth months of intrauterine life the testes normally begin to descend into a sac outside the body called the scrotum, an effect which may be controlled partly by the androgens produced by the fetal sex glands. The adult testes are therefore maintained in a temperature which is about 2°C lower than normal body temperature, a process which, some maintain, is necessary for normal spermatogenesis.

The adult testes are ovoid, approximately 4 cm long and 2 cm wide. The framework of each gland is provided by the fibrous tunica albuginea, the whole being surrounded by the serous tunica vaginalis. The walls of the coiled seminiferous tubules consist of several layers of spermatogenic cells with their supporting Sertoli cells, and the interstitial cells of Leydig form clumps between the tubules. The seminiferous tubules link up to form ducts which converge to form the convoluted duct of the epididymis. Arterial blood is supplied by the testicular artery; venous blood collects in a plexus which drains into the testicular vein. The right testicular vein drains into the inferior vena cava and the left into the left renal vein. The testis is also supplied with lymphatics which drain to para aortic nodes, and is innervated by sympathetic fibres. The nerve and vascular supplies enter and leave each testis via the spermatic cords. The capillaries in the testis have membranes which are not fenestrated.

Testicular hormones

Synthesis, storage, and release
The interstitial cells of Leydig synthesize, store, and secrete androgens (in particular testosterone) and small quantities of oestrogens. The various sex hormones are all steroids with 19 carbon atoms and are therefore often called the C-19 steroids (Chapter 4). Nearly all testosterone in the male is synthesized in the testes, less than 5 per cent being produced by the adrenals. The biosynthetic pathway is similar in both endocrine glands. The initial precursor molecule is cholesterol as for all steroid hormones. The testes, unlike the adrenals, only have the 17α-hydroxylase enzyme and not the 11β- and 21β-hydroxylases, with the result that pregnenolone formed from the cholesterol is hydroxylated only in position 17 of the molecule before being subjected to side-chain cleavage to form a ketosteroid. Some pregnenolone may alternatively be converted to progesterone which is then also hydroxylated before being converted to ketosteroid, although this pathway is not commonly followed in humans (see Fig. 5.2). Both ketosteroids are then converted to testosterone, which is the principal androgen secreted by the testes.

The normal daily secretion of testosterone in adult males is 4–9 mg. Once secreted, approximately 97–99 per cent of the testosterone is bound, either to plasma albumin or to a β-globulin which is specific for gonadal steroids (i.e. it also binds with oestrogens) and is therefore sometimes referred to as sex hormone binding globulin (SHBG). Total plasma levels of testosterone are approximately 13–30 nmol/l in adult men and 0·5–2·5 nmol/l in adult women.

Actions
In the adult male the testes have two important functions; the production of male gametes (spermatozoa) and the production of testosterone (and other less important androgens), and some oestrogen. The age at which the testes have developed sufficiently to perform these two functions so that reproduction is possible is known as puberty.

1. Spermatogenesis
The process leading to the formation of mature spermatozoa is called spermatogenesis, and takes place in the germinal epithelium of the seminiferous tubules. It consists of various stages, from the early spermatocyte to the spermatid to the mature spermatozoon. The Sertoli cells appear to be intimately involved in the maturation process. These cells contain high

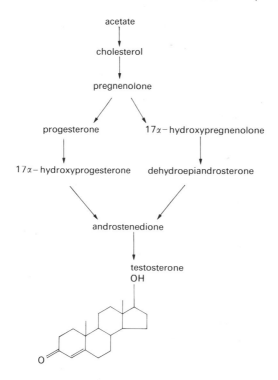

Fig.5.2   The biosynthesis pathways for testosterone from acetate.

concentrations of glycogen and probably have a nutritional, as well as a supportative, function. Ultrastructure studies have demonstrated that Sertoli cells enclose the germ cells at all stages of development.

2. *Testosterone production*

The various androgens (in particular testosterone) and the small quantities of oestrogens are secreted by the interstitial cells of Leydig. While the role of oestrogens in the function of the male reproductive tract is at present obscure, testosterone has various actions. In some tissues (e.g. skin, prostate), testosterone has to be converted to the more active dihydrotestosterone (DHT) by an enzyme, 5α-reductase, in order to exert its specific effects. However, this does not apply to all tissues and, for simplicity, the actions of DHT are not separated from testosterone; the situation is further complicated by the fact that DHT is also synthesized by the testes.

Testosterone stimulates the growth of the seminiferous tubules, and is an important regulator of spermatogenesis. In addition it is necessary for the development and maintenance of the accessory sex organs. These organs, which include the penis, the prostate, seminal vesicles, and bulbo-urethral glands, are usually defined as those organs which convey the gametes or add necessary constituents to the seminal fluid. In addition the scrotal capacity increases to accommodate the growing testes; the scrotum also becomes wrinkled and pigmented. The spermatozoa produced by the seminiferous tubules have very little cytoplasm of their own and therefore depend on the secretions of the accessory sex glands for nourishment. The seminal fluid is rich in fructose which is the source of metabolic energy for the spermatozoa, and is secreted by the seminal vesicles, in the form of a thick yellow fluid which forms the greater volume of the semen. The prostate gland secretes a thin fluid which is rich in calcium citrate, fibrinolysin, and acid phosphatase. The bulbo-urethral glands secrete mucus.

Testosterone is also necessary for the appearance and development of the secondary sex characteristics: these include the typical male physique, namely the muscular development and linear growth induced by stimulation of protein synthesis. Androgens are important anabolic agents, stimulating both cell growth and division. They stimulate epiphyseal growth, but also subsequently cause the epiphyses to fuse. The initial spurt of growth at puberty is therefore followed by its cessation. Testosterone induces the growth of facial and body hair, the recession of the scalp line, and the lowering of the voice pitch due to thickening of the vocal cords and enlargement of the larynx. While the development and maintenance of the male libido has in the past been believed to be due to androgens, the changes in behaviour which are often associated with the male, such as aggressive attitudes, may be only partly hormonal; social conditioning is probably an important factor. Nevertheless, exposure of the brain to testosterone during fetal development can lead to masculinization, an effect which may be due to intracellular oestrogens formed by intracellular aromatization of the testosterone. Other actions of androgens are to increase sebum secretion and to induce a mild retention of sodium, potassium, calcium, phosphate sulphate, and water by the kidneys.

Control of release

The production of testosterone in the adult male is controlled principally by luteinizing hormone (LH) from the adenohypophysis, which acts on the cells of Leydig and is therefore sometimes called interstitial-cell stimulating hormone (ICSH). The other adenohypophysial gonadotrophin, follicle-stimulating hormone (FSH) acts primarily on the seminiferous tubules to induce and maintain normal spermatogenesis. It is interesting to note, however, that there is some evidence which suggests that FSH may act synergistically with LH on steroidogenesis in the Leydig cells.

Castration is followed by increases in plasma gonadotrophin levels, which indicates that the testes normally have a negative feedback on the adenohypophysis or on the hypothalamus which secretes gonadotrophin-releasing factors (see Chapter 2). Testosterone is effective in reducing plasma LH levels, but only decreases FSH levels when the gonadal hormone is present in very large quantities. This strongly suggests that testosterone exerts a negative feedback on LH secretion, but that the release of FSH is controlled by some other factor from the testes. One substance that has been isolated from testicular extracts and which appears to inhibit FSH secretion has been called inhibin. This substance would appear to be secreted from the Sertoli cells in response to stimulation by FSH; the inhibin then exerts a negative feedback on

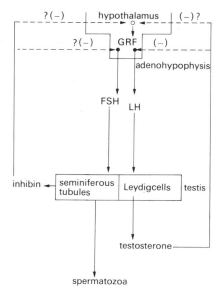

Fig.5.3   The possible negative feedback mechanisms involved in the stimulation of spermatogenesis by the seminiferous tubules and in the production of testosterone by the Leydig cells. The possible negative feedback loops by inhibin and testosterone on the hypothalamus would involve the release of the gonadotrophin releasing factor (GRF) which is probably FSH/LH RH.

FSH release. Thus the level of FSH in the male is controlled by the target hormone (Fig. 5.3).

The ovaries (oestrogens and progesterone)

Anatomy, histology, and development

From the sixth week of intrauterine life the embryonic gonads in genetic females develop into ovaries. The Mullerian duct system develops into Fallopian tubes and a uterus. In each ovary a cortex develops containing primordial follicles each of which consists of a germ cell surrounded by pregranulosa cells derived from the epithelium of the genital ridge. The theca interna and interstitial cells are derived from the mesoderm. During fetal life approximately 7 million germ cells develop, but many regress before birth so that at the time of birth about 200 000 oocytes are present. Of these cells, approximately 50 per cent regress at birth and the number of ova continues to decrease until puberty when only a few hundred remain. Meiosis of the oocyte, which begins *in utero*, is arrested at the first prophase until ovulation when the first meiotic division occurs. The second meiotic division is stimulated when fertilization takes place.

The two ovaries are ovoid glands, one on each side of the uterus. Nerves, blood vessels, and lymphatics penetrate the ovary at the hilum of the gland.

The arterial supply arises from the aorta while the venous drainage leaves the hilum in the pampiniform plexus to form the ovarian veins. The right ovarian vein drains into the inferior vena cava while the left vein drains into the left renal vein. Each ovary consists of three regions, the outer cortex, the inner medulla, and a hilum around the point of attachment to its mesentery. The follicles are located in the stroma of the cortex, and a number mature with each ovarian cycle.

Oestrogens

Synthesis, storage, and release

While the developing ovaries in the fetus may not produce hormones, the theca interna cells of the follicles in the adult ovaries synthesize oestrogens. These hormones are C-19 steroids, the major one to be secreted being 17β-oestradiol. Other sites of oestrogen production are the corpus luteum, the feto-placental unit and, to a minor extent, the adrenal cortex.

The biosynthesis of oestrogens involves the formation of androgens from pregnenolone. Once it is released into the circulation, some oestradiol is metabolized to oestrone with which it is in equilibrium. The oestrone, which is less potent than oestradiol, may then be further metabolized to another, even less potent, oestrogen called oestriol (see Fig. 5.4). The oestrogens are mostly (70 per cent) bound to plasma proteins, principally sex hormone binding globulin (SHBG) which also binds testosterone. Oestradiol is metabolized to various substances which are excreted in human urine. The plasma oestrogen concentrations vary throughout the menstrual cycle being of the order of 0·075–0·2 nmol/l during the follicular phase, reaching peak levels of 0·35–1·5 nmol/l just before ovulation; the levels then decrease before rising to a second peak of 0·2–1·1 nmol/l at the mid-point of the secretory phase.

Actions

Oestrogens are necessary for the development and maintenance of the uterus, the Fallopian tubes, the cervix, the vagina, the labia minora and majora, and the breasts. The role of oestrogens in the growth and development of the uterine endometrium during the proliferative phase of the menstrual cycle will be discussed subsequently. Oestrogens increase both the motility of the Fallopian tubes and the excitability of uterine muscle. During pregnancy, oestrogens stimulate myometrial growth by increasing the glycogen and actinomyosin content of the muscle, and sensitize it to the stimulatory actions of oxytocin, possibly by altering the availability of free calcium ions. Oestrogens act on the cervical mucosa making the mucus thinner and more alkaline, both changes favouring the survival and transport of spermatozoa after coitus. At ovulation the mucus is thinnest and if a cervical smear is made, a fern-like pattern can be seen (see clinical section of this chapter). Oestrogens also cause changes in vaginal cytology, inducing cornification of the epithelium. During pregnancy the proliferation of the mammary ducts in preparation for lactation is stimulated by oestrogens. Feminine secondary sex characteristics such as broad hips, the accumulation of fat in the breasts and buttocks, and the high ratio of scalp to body hair depend on oestrogens acting in the absence of large amounts of circulating androgens. Nevertheless it is

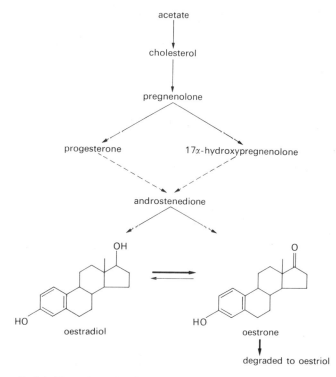

Fig.5.4 The pathways involved in the synthesis of oestradiol and oestrone.

quite possible that androgens as well as oestrogens act on the central nervous system and that both groups of hormones contribute to the maintenance of sexual libido in women.

Other effects of oestrogens include mild salt and water retention which in normal women may be associated with an increased body weight just before menstruation. This may contribute to the irritability and tension associated with 'premenstrual tension'. Finally oestrogens decrease circulating plasma cholesterol levels by a mechanism which has not yet been completely eluci-dated, but may involve an action on the lipoproteins associated with the cholesterol. This may be one of the factors responsible for the lower incidence of arteriosclerosis recorded in women.

Progesterone

Synthesis, storage, and release

Progesterone is a C-21 steroid which is an important intermediate in the synthesis of steroid hormones in all tissues that secrete them. Progesterone itself is secreted primarily by the corpus luteum and the placenta, but also to a small extent by the adrenal cortex and the testes. One derivative, 17α-hydroxyprogesterone, appears to be secreted with oestrogens by the ovarian follicles. Little is known concerning the precise mechanism of release of progesterone or of its transport in the blood, although it is probably mostly bound to plasma proteins. It has a short half-life of approximately 5 minutes in the blood, and is converted to pregnanediol mainly in the liver, and subsequently conjugated with glucuronic acid; it is excreted in the urine chiefly in the form of the glucoronide.

During the follicular (proliferative) phase of the menstrual cycle, the normal plasma progesterone level is less than 5 nmol/l. During the luteal (secretory) phase, the level rises to peak values of 40–50 nmol/l due to the much greater quantities of progesterone produced by the maintained corpus luteum. In men the normal plasma progesterone level is of the order of 1·0 nmol/l.

Actions

As will be mentioned in the brief discussion on the menstrual cycle, progesterone is responsible for the secretory (progestational) changes in the endometrium. The cervical mucus becomes thick and cellular, and the mucous secretion from the vaginal walls is also thickened. The effect of progesterone on the myometrium is antagonistic to oestrogen so that the excitability of the individual cells decreases, as does their sensitivity to oxytocin. It increases the cellular membrane potential and decreases the spontaneous electrical activity. The development of the lobules and alveoli of the mammary tissue in the breasts is also stimulated by progesterone.

Other effects of this hormone include a rise in basal metabolic rate and body temperature, and stimulation of respiration. In large doses it appears to induce a natriuresis, possibly by inhibiting the action of circulating aldosterone.

The menstrual cycle

In order to understand the endocrine function of the ovaries it is necessary to consider the regular cyclic changes which occur from puberty to the menopause. These cyclic changes are called menstrual cycles in the higher primates, each of which lasts for 28 days on average, although the actual length of the cycle may vary considerably. This regular pattern can be considered as a periodic preparation of the adult female for fertilization and pregnancy.

1. Ovarian changes

At the beginning of each cycle some ovarian follicles start to grow rapidly under the influence of gonadotrophins, while those of the preceeding cycle regress. A maturing follicle is called a Graafian follicle and is composed of follicular fluid containing a germ cell (an ovum) surrounded by two principal layers of cells: the inner granulosa cells and the outer theca interna cells. The theca interna cells secrete the female sex hormones, the oestrogens. One follicle continues to grow until it ruptures and the ovum is extruded into the abdominal cavity (ovulation). The ovum is trapped by the specialized endings of the Fallopian tubes and transported to the uterus where it becomes implanted if fertilization occurs. Those follicles which enlarge but fail to ovulate, degenerate. At ovulation the follicle fills with blood (the corpus haemorrhagicum). The granulosa and theca interna cells lining the follicle then proliferate until the blood is replaced by luteal cells forming the corpus luteum. The luteal cells contain relatively high concentrations of lipids and are the sites of synthesis not only of progesterone but also oestrogens. If pregnancy occurs the corpus luteum persists and continues to secrete progesterone and oestrogens, although after about the third month the feto-placental unit (see later) assumes this function. If pregnancy fails to occur the corpus luteum degenerates and a new menstrual cycle begins.

2. Uterine changes

By convention, the first day of each menstrual cycle is considered as the first day of menstruation when the developed endometrium starts to be shed. By about the fifth day menstruation ceases and the oestrogens from the developing ovarian follicles cause the endometrium to proliferate again and uterine glands to develop (proliferative phase). This continues until ovulation (approximately day 14), when the progesterone now induces coiling and folding of the various secretory glands and their blood-vessels in the endometrium. The glands are stimulated to secrete a glycogen-rich watery mucus by the action of increasing levels of progesterone from the corpus luteum (the secretory phase).

This secretory phase is maintained until around day 28 when menstruation begins if pregnancy has not occurred. The spiral arteries within the endometrium which developed during the proliferative phase constrict causing ischaemia of the endometrium. They then dilate and their necrotic walls rupture producing haemorrhage and sloughing. Blood shed in the uterus clots and is subsequently liquefied by enzymes. Menstruation is the most obvious physical characteristic of the cycle and is initiated by the withdrawal of hormonal support from the corpus luteum as this regresses. The bleeding ends when the spiral arteries again constrict after approximately 5 days, followed by regeneration of a new endometrium. The rise in progesterone levels just before ovulation induces a slight increase in the basal body temperature, a response which may result partly from a direct effect of this hormone on the hypothalamic thermo-regulatory centre. The daily measurement of the basal body temperature can therefore be used as an indicator of ovarian progesterone production and may detect the time of ovulation.

Control of ovarian hormone secretion

The menstrual cycle is associated with the differential secretion of oestrogens and progesterone which is, in turn, related to the release of gonadotrophic hormones from the adenohypophysis.

For some time it was generally believed that the periodic changes of the menstrual cycle were regulated by the adenohypophysial gonadotrophins, their release being mainly controlled by an inherent rhythmicity of the hypothalamus. It is now reasonably certain however that the changes of the menstrual cycle are regulated by means of a much more complicated system involving a fine balance between gonadotrophins and gonadal hormones through positive and negative feedback mechanisms, nervous influences from other parts of the brain to the hypothalamus and intra-ovarian mechanisms.

Furthermore, the sensitivity of the hypothalamic–pituitary system can actually be altered by the circulating levels of oestrogens in the blood such that if low levels are present, the sensitivity of the system to a sudden small increase in oestrogen concentration is enhanced. These various controlling influences are considered in the following discussion of the hormonal control of the menstrual cycle.

Hormonal control

During and following menstruation, in the follicular phase of the cycle, the low level of circulating oestrogens results in an increase in the secretion of FSH which stimulates follicular development in the presence of basal quantities of circulating LH. Growth of the follicles is associated with an increased secretion of oestrogens and circulating levels rise accordingly. There is evidence to suggest that the oestrogens have an intra-ovarian action which directly influences follicular growth as well as to increase the responsiveness of the ovaries to the circulating gonadotrophins. Androgens appear to inhibit these effects. As the level of circulating oestradiol increases during the late follicular phase of the cycle it has a further positive feedback effect on FSH and LH release. By the thirteenth day circulating levels of LH increase sharply reaching peak values after the maximal level of circulating oestradiol has been achieved. This surge of LH secretion, which is accompanied by a rise in FSH, is due to the positive feedback by oestradiol. The combination of gonadotrophins brings about the final maturation of the Graafian follicle and ovulation. The high levels of oestradiol apparently now act to inhibit the release of the gonadotrophins. Subsequently the plasma levels of oestradiol fall. The secretory activity of the corpus luteum then leads to an increased secretion of progesterone and to a second rise in the circulating oestradiol level, both circulating hormone concentrations reaching a peak at about the same time. Basal levels of LH appear to be necessary for the maintenance of luteal function. After approximately 14 days, if fertilization has not occurred, the corpus luteum regresses perhaps because of the local accumulation of a critical quantity of oestrogens. Regression of the corpus luteum results in a fall in circulating oestrogen and progesterone concentrations and leads to menstruation and the beginning of a new cycle (Fig. 5.5).

It is important to emphasize that the outline of the hormonal control of the menstrual cycle outlined above is a gross simplification. Many points require confirmation while others remain controversial. For example, the precise circumstances under which oestrogens exert a positive or a negative feedback effect on gonadotrophin secretion are uncertain. Furthermore, it is not yet confirmed that there is a single hypothalamic releasing hormone for both FSH and LH. The independent secretion of either gonadotrophin may depend on the actions of the relative initial concentrations of circulating gonadal and adrenal hormones on the hypothalamus and adenohypophysis. Steroid hormones can induce changes in hypothalamic stores of the decapeptide LHRH, in the responsiveness of the adenohypophysial cells to the releasing hormone, and in the availability of trophic hormones for immediate release into the circulation. It is quite possible that releasing-hormones other than LHRH may interact with the factors outlined above. It is therefore important to appreciate

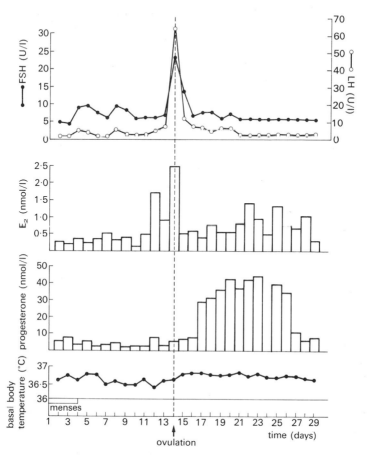

Fig.5.5 The typical pattern of changes in plasma concentrations of follicle stimulating hormone (FSH), luteinizing hormone (LH), oestradiol (E_2), and progesterone, and in the basal body temperature in a woman with normal ovulatory menstrual cycles. The Figure is reproduced by kind permission of the Academic Press, and the authors from an article by Vande Wiele *et al.* entitled 'Mechanisms regulating the menstrual cycle in women' in *Rec. Prog. Horm. Res.* (1970) **26**, 76.

the apparent complexity of the control of adenohypophysial function with respect to gonadotrophin release. This is not a unique situation since the secretion of other hormones, such as insulin, is controlled by equally complex systems involving changes in the responsiveness of the cells by modulating factors. In each case the complexity of the control system allows for greater adaptability in response to particular stimuli.

For the role of oestrogen and progesterone as oral contraceptives, see pp. 101–2.

Pregnancy

After conception, the corpus luteum continues to produce progesterone which maintains the endometrium in the 'progestational' state essential for pregnancy. The implanting blastocyst secretes human chorionic gonadotrophin (HCG) which maintains luteal function for approximately 8 weeks. The placenta gradually takes over steroid production from the corpus luteum and by the twelfth week has usually become the principal site of progesterone and oestrogen synthesis. Placental steroids are synthesized from precursors derived from the fetus. The maternal adrenal glands also contribute to the total progesterone production. Progesterone and oestrogen concentrations continue to increase in the maternal circulation throughout pregnancy, and inhibit the release of maternal gonadotrophins. The principal urinary excretory products are oestriol and pregnanediol which arise from conversions in both maternal and fetal tissues. The important functions of the feto-placental unit are discussed in the following section.

In late pregnancy, the maternal blood oestrogen level appears to follow a circadian rhythm, being lowest in the afternoon around 4.30 p.m. Oestrogen (and progesterone) production in pregnancy is controlled partly by the placental hormone HCG, although other factors are probably involved.

During pregnancy many other endocrine glands are affected. The adenohypophysis is enlarged and there is an increase in the secretion of corticotrophin, thyrotrophin, and somatotrophin, while, as described previously, gonadotrophin release is inhibited by the large quantities of circulating oestrogen and progesterone. Adrenal corticosteroid production increases throughout pregnancy to reach a peak level at parturition. Since plasma protein synthesis is increased during pregnancy it was originally believed that the increase in total cortisol levels resulted from the increase in the protein-bound cortisol. However it now appears that the free-cortisol component also increases some threefold in late pregnancy. The physiological effects of increased cortisol levels during pregnancy remain obscure. Aldosterone production is increased, and this together with the renal effects of oestrogens cause increased sodium reabsorption from the renal tubule, and hence a fluid retention.

The thyroid gland may enlarge by approximately 50 per cent during pregnancy as a result of increased thyrotrophin secretion, but only the total thyroxine concentration is raised, due to increased protein binding, and hyperthyroidism does not occur. The parathyroid glands also often increase in size and activity, possibly induced by the increasing requirements for calcium by the growing fetus. Increased quantities of parathormone are believed to be secreted to maintain the maternal calcium level by mobilizing bone calcium, enhancing the absorption of calcium from the gastrointestinal tract (through its action on vitamin D metabolism) and decreasing its renal excretion (see Chapter 7).

Finally, a polypeptide called relaxin isolated from the corpora lutea of the ovaries is also claimed to have a role in pregnancy especially at parturition. It is believed to cause the relaxation of the ligaments of the symphysis pubis (also induced by oestrogens and progesterone), a softening of the cervix at the time of delivery and to inhibit uterine motility. Whether these possible effects of relaxin aid the passage of the fetus at parturition is debatable.

Feto-placental unit

All mammals are viviparous (with the exception of the spiny anteater and the duck-billed platypus). It is, therefore, essential that some portion of the embryo establishes a connection with the maternal structures, in order to acquire oxygen and nutritional substances necessary for development, and to enable the disposal of the end products of metabolism. This essential structure is the placenta.

In placental mammals, the ovarian cycle is shorter than the gestation period. This has led to the evolutionary development in pregnancy of a trophoblast able to synthesize hormones which, in conjunction with the fetus, forms a complex endocrine structure. The trophoblast consists of an inner cellular layer called the cytotrophoblast (Langhan's layer) and an outer syncytiotrophoblast, which is in direct contact with maternal blood.

After fertilization the ovarian secretion of oestrogen and progesterone prepares the endometrium for implantation of the blastocyst. The effect of the ovarian corpus luteum wanes after the early weeks of pregnancy, when the placenta takes over the hormonal responsibility. The feto-placental unit is primarily responsible for oestrogen production, but is also responsible for the synthesis of progesterone, human placental lactogen (HPL), and HCG. There is evidence that the placenta also synthesizes human chorionic thyrotrophin which has a similar action to TSH, but is antigenically slightly different. The high levels of prolactin in amniotic fluid suggest that the placenta may manufacture this hormone. The placenta may also produce other polypeptide hormones, but confirmation of this does not yet exist.

The site of production of the steroid hormones in the placenta appears to be the syncytium, although this has not been established. Fluorescent antibody studies have demonstrated the presence of HCG in the syncytium and not in the cytotrophoblast, but this may indicate the site of storage rather than synthesis. However, the rate of production of HCG appears to correlate more with the volume of the cytotrophoblast than of the syncytium.

Human chorionic gonadotrophin

This is a glycoprotein similar to LH. It is only found in the presence of the trophoblast and indeed its measurement is used as a marker in monitoring the treatment of trophoblastic disease. Detection of HCG in the urine forms the basis of the immunological pregnancy test which becomes positive approximately 28 days after conception. The recent development of a radioimmuno assay to detect the presence of a subunit of HCG in maternal serum now allows diagnosis of pregnancy even before the first missed period.

The secretion of HCG begins soon after fertilization, and its level reaches a peak about 50–60 days after the last menstrual bleed. The concentration then falls dramatically over 10 days to a new level which remains constant until the end of pregnancy. A second small increase is observed between the twenty-eighth and thirty-sixth weeks.

The role of HCG may be regarded as one of bridging the gap between ovarian maintenance of pregnancy and the established pregnant state. It is widely accepted that HCG is luteotrophic and maintains the corpus luteum until the placenta becomes endocrinologically autonomous. High levels of

HCG can be demonstrated after the corpus luteum atrophies and this suggests that the hormone has other functions which remain obscure. It appears to stimulate the fetal production of dehydroepiandrosterone (DHEA) which is then converted to oestrogens by the placenta. In the male fetus HCG stimulates the interstitial cells of Leydig which begin to secrete testosterone. The small quantities of testosterone produced at this stage are involved in stimulating the development of the male sex organs.

Human placental lactogen

This can be detected in maternal serum by the sixth week of gestation (with little crossing the placenta to reach the fetus). Immunofluorescent studies suggest that the syncytium is involved in its synthesis. The levels of HPL rise steadily throughout pregnancy, the curve flattening off towards term. Falling levels of HPL during early pregnancy suggest that abortion may be inevitable, or if occurring later indicate placental insufficiency. The hormone is structurally very similar to somatotrophin and has many of its biological and immunological properties.

The exact endocrine role of HPL in pregnancy is not yet known. It exhibits several different actions including lactogenic and growth promoting properties; mammotrophic and luteotrophic properties have also been described. HPL has a lipolytic action and may provide an alternative source of energy to glycogenolysis. The anti-insulin effect of HPL may be responsible for the diabetogenic changes of pregnancy. The control of its secretion is likewise poorly understood, but since its production appears to be related to placental (and hence fetal) weight its measurement serves as a valuable indicator of the condition of the fetus. It may be that in some way HPL and perhaps HCG protect the fetus from rejection by the mother.

Oestrogens

The ovary is the only endocrine gland which can synthesize oestrogens from acetate. However, the placenta possesses a very powerful aromatizing system which is capable of converting C-19 steroids into oestrogens. The fetal and maternal adrenal cortex both synthesize large quantities of dehydroepiandrosterone sulphate, and it is mainly this which is converted to oestrogens in the placenta.

Very much more oestriol is produced by the placenta than the other two oestrogens, oestrone and 17β-oestradiol. Approximately half is derived from maternal adrenal precursors and half from fetal adrenal precursors.

The measurement of oestriol in 24-h urine specimens is used to assess the function of the feto-placental unit in pregnancy. Where fetal function is affected, a relatively greater fall of oestriol levels is observed than of those hormones synthesized solely by the placenta. Urinary oestriol excretion thus reflects both placental function and fetal well-being.

Progesterone

Large amounts of progesterone are formed in the placenta in the later stages of pregnancy. Unlike oestrogen, progesterone can be synthesized in the placenta from acetate or cholesterol. Its measurement, either as plasma progesterone or as urinary pregnenediol, is thought to reflect pure placental function.

Parturition

Uterine contractility is inhibited by progesterone during pregnancy. Progesterone is secreted in steadily increasing quantities as the pregnancy approaches term, together with oestrogen. Oestrogens increase the state of uterine contractility, and as pregnancy progresses the oestrogen levels rise to a relatively greater extent than progesterone so that the uterus becomes gradually oestrogen-dominated. Just before term, it is believed that the oestrogen to progesterone ratio is such that the uterine smooth muscle becomes particularly sensitive to the neurohypophysial hormone oxytocin which may stimulate uterine contractions. Oxytocin is probably released in spurts from the neurohypophysis through the mediation of a neurogenic reflex as the cervix is stretched due to uterine contractions.

In addition, as the cervix dilates it may elicit uterine contractions directly, either through a nervous or myogenic reflex. The periodic contractions of labour become progressively stronger, possibly because of one of the above positive feedback mechanisms. It must be appreciated that this account only applies to established labour and the factor or factors responsible for the initiation of labour are still unknown. Furthermore, while oxytocin is used therapeutically to induce parturition its physiological role in this process remains uncertain.

Lactation

The production of milk is the chief function of the breasts. In the female the breasts develop at puberty, but normally become functional only at parturition. Various hormones are involved in developing and maintaining the breasts, including the gonadal hormones oestrogen and progesterone and the adenohypophysial gonadotrophins and prolactin. As described previously oestrogen stimulates the development of the duct system in the breast while progesterone stimulates growth of the alveoli. However, growth hormone and adrenocorticosteroids also appear to be necessary for the full development of the duct system, and prolactin is required for the complete development of the alveolar lobules. During pregnancy oestrogen, progesterone, and HPL are produced by the placenta in large quantities and it is chiefly in response to these hormones that the breasts fully develop at this stage. Delivery of the child results in an immediate decrease in progesterone levels following the loss of the placenta; the oestrogen concentration also decreases, but less dramatically. This withdrawal of placental hormones results in hormonal domination of the breasts by prolactin which, in the presence of insulin, adrenal corticosteroids, and thyroid hormones initiates the secretion of milk into the duct system. Release of prolactin is believed to be due partly to an inhibition of the release of the hypothalamic inhibitory factor, but also may be due to the stimulating of a hypothalamic releasing-factor. Milk will not flow out of the ducts to the nipple unless suckling takes place. If this occurs, the tactile stimulation of the nipple results in a neuro-endocrine reflex release of the neurohypophysial hormone oxytocin which acts by stimulating contraction of the myoepithelial cells surrounding the alveoli, and the smooth muscle of the ductile system. Milk is forced into the main ducts of the breast which ultimately connect to the nipple so that milk ejection can take place. The plasma basal concentrations of prolactin decrease after birth. However suckling has been found to stimulate the release not only of oxytocin but also of prolactin. Hence neuroendocrine reflexes are responsible for the secretion of both hormones; an ideal situation in that the secretion and expulsion of milk from the lactating breasts occur together.

CLINICAL DISORDERS OF THE MALE

Disorders of the male resulting from a low blood concentration of testosterone may be either primary (testicular malfunction) or secondary (impaired secretion of trophic hormones); in addition, the target tissue may be insensitive to the normal levels of testicular hormone. Even though the genital changes can be marked the patient may only be concerned with the failure to conceive (infertility) and/or the inability to copulate. It is often assumed that infertility is only due to a failure to produce an adequate number of spermatozoa, but it may be due to other, ill-understood factors, such as lack of 'mental rest'. 'Antagonistic secretions' of the female genital tract which prevent fertilization, or even inadequate knowledge of the anatomy of the female external genitals may also be responsible. Failure of copulation is due either to the inability to achieve an erection (impotence) and/or the lack of sexual desire (diminished libido). It must be emphasized that both of these may occur in general metabolic disorders such as diabetes mellitus or in psychological disturbances.

Hypersecretion of androgens is considered in the section on sexual precocity. This section briefly considers the conditions of testicular deficiency, some testicular disorders, and infertility.

Testosterone disorders

Excess

No such disorders are known.

Deficiency

A failure in the development of the primary sex glands results in lack of testosterone with a consequently impaired development of the accessory sex organs and secondary sex characters, and in infertility.

If there is a deficiency or absence of testosterone in the young, puberty is delayed and bone age retarded. If untreated the typical eunuchoid pattern may be seen.

The patient is generally tall with long limbs (arm span greater than height, and leg length exceeds that of the trunk). The skin is usually pale and fine. Pubic and axillary hair is absent or scanty, and the facial hair is fine; sometimes the patient never shaves or does so only in order to conform. Muscle development is poor and power is limited. The voice has the high pitch associated with that of a woman. The genitals are immature; the testicles and penis are small, while the scrotum lacks its natural rugosity.

1. Seminiferous tubule dysgenesis (Klinefelter's syndrome)
This is an example of primary testicular failure associated with a chromosome abnormality; there are 47 chromosomes due to an additional X-chromosome (XXY). The standard buccal smear will therefore reveal positive Barr bodies on the microscopic examination.

CLINICAL FEATURES: The clinical features are variable. Usually the testes are small, relatively insensitive, and firmer than normal; frequently the penis is small, but the secondary sex characteristics range from almost normal to the full eunuchoid state. Gynaecomastia, though at one time claimed to be a characteristic feature, may not be present; sometimes there is unilateral breast development. It is interesting to note that intelligence is frequently impaired and there may be behavioural problems. The patient is infertile and both the sexual desire and the ability to have erections are impaired. Clinically, it may be difficult to distinguish seminiferous tubule dysgenesis from post mumps orchitis.

Klinefelter's syndrome is the most common genetically determined testicular defect. Various subclinical types of the syndrome may be associated with mosaicism (genotype varies in different parts of the body). There are other rare forms of chromosome abnormalities associated with hypogonadism.

INVESTIGATIONS:

1. A buccal smear is the first test followed, if possible, by karyotyping. The former will reveal Barr bodies and the latter will show an extra X-chromosome. This chromosomal abnormality is found in the majority of patients with this syndrome. Less severe changes may occur with mosaicism.

2. The blood concentration of trophic hormones and testosterone are estimated. Typically the blood concentration of FSH is elevated and frequently the LH is also raised, but this will depend on the blood-level of testosterone.

3. It is claimed that the histological changes of the testes such as hyalinization of the basement membrane of the tubular cells, which are largely replaced by Sertoli cells, are characteristic of the condition. The interstitial cells are reduced in number, and as expected there is impaired spermatogenesis.

TREATMENT: Testosterone propionate (Testoral) is administered 10 mg sublingually three times a day while testosterone as Sustenon is administered in a dose of 250 mg once or twice monthly.

2. Testicular feminization syndrome
It is believed that in this condition there is a failure of the appropriate cells of the body to respond to testosterone.

CLINICAL FEATURES: The genotype is usually recorded as female at birth because of the genitalia. Although there is an introitus (a small passage which ends blindly) the uterus, Fallopian tubes, and ovaries are absent; sometimes the clitoris is larger than normal. Breast development may be normal (female). These patients may not present until puberty with amenorrhoea, and/or scanty, or absent, pubic or axillary hair. Sometimes these patients are seen after marriage at infertility clinics.

The testes may be intra-abdominal or anywhere along the inguinal canal; indeed it is sometimes possible to palpate one or both testes in the 'labia'.

INVESTIGATIONS: The patient is genotyped. Blood concentration of trophic hormones and testosterone are measured. The hormone concentrations are normal and the genotype is male.

TREATMENT: While the genetic pattern is male, mentality is female. The testes are surgically removed because of the possibility of malignant change and oestrogens are given in some convenient form, for example, ethinyl oestradiol, about 20 μg/24h to prevent menopausal symptoms.

3. Severe bilateral orchitis

This is a well-recognized complication of mumps in young men (incidence about 20 per cent).

CLINICAL FEATURES: The testes become tender and swollen, usually a few days after the swelling of the parotid gland(s). In the adult infertility may be a consequence and on rare occasions when the orchitis occurs before puberty not only may there be infertility but also hypogonadism. Orchitis may also be a complication of infection with varicella-zoster or the Coxsachie virus; it may also be a complication of congenital syphilis.

INVESTIGATIONS: If infertility and hypogonadism are present, the investigations are the same as for seminiferous tubule dysgenesis.

TREATMENT: During the acute phase corticoid therapy may be of benefit, but this therapy does not reduce the incidence of infertility. If there is eunuchoidism, androgen therapy is given (see seminiferous tubule dysgenesis).

4. Secondary testicular degeneration

This is a consequence of a lesion in the hypothalamic–adenohypophysial system. This may be due to tumours of the adenohypophysis (sarcoid or metastatic invasion) or sometimes it may be due to an isolated failure of gonadotrophic secretion.

CLINICAL FEATURES: These are eunuchoid changes (see primary lesion), but in addition there may be alterations associated with a deficiency of the other trophic hormones.

INVESTIGATIONS: The blood concentrations of the trophic hormones are determined and characteristically there are low levels of gonadotrophins; sometimes the other trophic hormones are also decreased.

TREATMENT: Androgens are administered as described previously.

Other disorders

Finally three specific testicular disorders are considered.

1. Undescended testicle (cryptorchidism)

While bilateral undescended testicles are usually associated with infertility there may be no endocrine abnormality.

The testes normally enter the scrotum by the seventh month of intrauterine life. However, pathological processes may prevent the gubernacular testes from performing their normal action. If at birth both testes are absent from the scrotal sac, they will descend in most babies by the end of the first year. It is sometimes extremely difficult to differentiate an undescended testicle from the retractile type in the young. However, by careful palpation the retractile testes can be placed into the correct position if the hands are warm and the child is in a warm bath.

The undescended testicle may be in any position along the normal route of descent and may occasionally be in an abnormal site (ectopic); a congenitally abnormal testicle may fail to descend. Fortunately the effect is commonly unilateral and only in the undescended testicle may spermatogenesis be adversely affected, apparently because of the higher environmental temperature.

TREATMENT: This is a problem, not only with respect to when to begin treatment, but also whether surgery or hormonal therapy should be employed. Possibly the best therapy is to give chorionic gonadotrophin 400 IU thrice weekly in the early years. If the testicles have not descended by about the seventh year, surgery is indicated. The testicle is placed in the scrotal sac even though subsequently it may fail to produce spermatozoa, because an undescended testicle may undergo malignant change. It is possible that the treatment of this condition may in the future be LHRH.

2. Malignant tumours of the testicle

These tumours may secrete oestrogens or androgens and produce symptoms of hypersecretion (see precocious sexual puberty). They may be primary germinal (seminoma or teratoma) non-germinal (interstitial or Sertolic cells), or due to a malignant deposit from a tumour elsewhere.

CLINICAL FEATURES: Usually the tumours present as painless swellings of the testes and there may be metastases in the regional lymph nodes.

INVESTIGATIONS: Blood levels of oestrogens and androgens are determined.

TREATMENT: Surgical removal is the primary treatment, followed if required by radiation therapy.

3. Torsion of the testicle

This may occur without a history of trauma. There is an acute, painful swelling of the testicle and it may occupy an abnormal position. This is treated surgically.

Infertility

Even in the absence of disease in either partner, infertility may be as high as 10 per cent. Oligospermia or azoospermia may be due to organic damage of the tubular system of the testes or to insufficiency of testosterone. Recently it has been found that some infertile patients may have antibodies to spermatozoa. It is valuable to assess whether in the past the patient has been fertile. It may appear unnecessary, but it should be confirmed that full sexual intercourse is occurring.

There is a general examination of the patient followed by a careful examination of the genitals. The size, consistency, and the degree of tenderness of the testicles are determined. Abnormalities of the vas deferens should be excluded. Varicocoels of the testes are frequently associated with infertility. The normal size of the flaccid penis is extremely variable and is of no diagnostic value. The chest wall should be examined for any true enlargement of the breast; body hair distribution is noted.

INVESTIGATIONS: Routine tests are carried out to exclude general metabolic disorders; for example, full blood-count, erythrocyte sedimentation rate (ESR), chest X-ray, blood-glucose. The normal sperm-count is 100×10^6/ml; at $20-40 \times 10^6$/ml about 50 per cent are sterile and if below 20×10^6/ml the patient is sterile. If the count is below normal the blood concentration of the gonadotrophic hormones and testosterone are determined.

TREATMENT: Infertility in the male (excluding those cases due to general metabolic disorders) is extremely difficult to treat successfully. Occasionally there have been claims that gonadotrophic hormones and/or Clomiphene induce fertility (see p. 97).

Artificial insemination and other techniques are not considered in this book.

Impotence

Impotence occurs in the eunuchoid state but sometimes the patient may claim that his libido is unaltered. While metabolic disorders such as diabetes mellitus, and general debilitating disorders (e.g. tuberculosis) may cause a loss of sexual potency it is rarely a primary complaint. The type of impotence considered here is the condition in which it is the presenting symptom. In the past if there was no evidence of testicular malfunction, chronic disease, or metabolic disorder the condition was considered to be psychological in origin. The treatment of these patients was difficult and testosterone therapy was often advocated probably because of the psychological effect on the patient of receiving an androgen. It has been found however, that some of these patients have high plasma prolactin levels and bromocriptine therapy has been used with good results.

The treatment of those patients who have normal plasma prolactin levels is still difficult. In this situation it is essential to establish that the complaint is real and if it is they should be referred to a psychosexual unit for guidance.

CLINICAL DISORDERS OF THE FEMALE

Unlike the clinical disorders of other endocrine glands, disorders of the ovary are not classified here as deficient or excess secretion of ovarian hormones.

Instead, the classification followed in this chapter, although arbitrary, allows for a consideration of those common female disabilities which are not readily divided into hypo- or hyper-secretion conditions. Furthermore, these disorders may to some extent be due to the malfunction of another endocrine gland. The necessity for using this different system does however emphasize the individuality of this sex.

The commonest endocrine disorder of the female is some disturbance of the menstrual cycle, but whether this disturbance is abnormal may be difficult to determine. The normal range may extend from a regular cycle of around 28 days to very infrequent menstrual bleeds every few months, (oligomenorrhoea) or even very occasionally to amenorrhoea (absent menstruation); the effect of emotional factors on this rhythm is well recognized (see Fig. 5.6). Naturally, associated with amenorrhoea is infertility, namely failure of ovulation. This, being the most important disorder, is considered first. Other conditions which are considered in subsequent sections are premenstrual tension, metropathia haemorrhagica, hirsutism, and the rare conditions of hormone-secreting ovarian tumours. Also discussed in this section are two related topics, the menopause and the contraceptive pill.

Ovulation and the failure to ovulate

Clinically normal ovulation encompasses a wide spectrum from the regularly ovulating female at one end, to the patient with prolonged secondary amenorrhoea at the other.

INVESTIGATIONS: It is difficult to be certain on clinical grounds that ovulation is occurring. The only absolute proof of ovulation is pregnancy, but there are other observations and routine investigations which may help in the assessment. These observations and investigations are:

1. *The history of the menstrual cycle.* A regular cycle and dysmenorrhoea suggest that ovulation is occurring. Conversely the woman with amenorrhoea is unlikely to be ovulating, although should this occur and fertilization is successful, it can cause considerable confusion in calculating the length of gestation. Sometimes women notice lower abdominal pain for a brief period at ovulation (Mittleschmerz).

2. *Basal temperature chart.* The body temperature dips and then rises at the time of ovulation. This is thought to be an effect of progesterone. This temperature change is used to time ovulation, in retrospect, in both those who want to conceive and those who do not.

3. *Measurement of progesterone levels.* A plasma progesterone level of 10 nmol/l or more, 7 days before menstruation (i.e. 7 days after ovulation) indicates the formation of a corpus luteum, although the range in the luteal phase is 5–60 nmol/l. Urinary pregnanediol is also increased this being an end-product of progesterone metabolism and is easily measured. The plasma progesterone level is nevertheless the most reliable test.

4. *Vaginal smears.* A vaginal smear is easily obtained even in a virgin and on histological examination will reveal characteristic changes if there is sufficient progesterone.

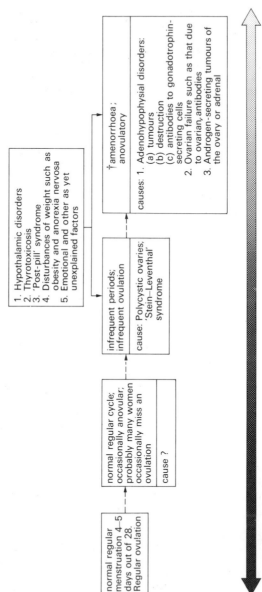

normal regular
menstruation 4–5
days out of 28.
Regular ovulation

cause ?

normal regular cycle;
occasionally anovular;
probably many women
occasionally miss an
ovulation

infrequent periods;
infrequent ovulation

cause: Polycystic ovaries;
'Stein–Leventhal'
syndrome

1. Hypothalamic disorders
2. Thyrotoxicosis
3. 'Post-pill' syndrome
4. Disturbances of weight such as
   obesity and anorexia nervosa
5. Emotional and other as yet
   unexplained factors

†amenorrhoea;
anovulatory

causes: 1. Adenohypophysial disorders:
          (a) tumours
          (b) destruction
          (c) antibodies to gonadotrophin-
              secreting cells
       2. Ovarian failure such as that due
          to ovarian, antibodies
       3. Androgen-secreting tumours of
          the ovary or adrenal

†Excluded from the table are physiological causes of amenorrhoea such as pregnancy, lactation, and the menopause; also excluded are general metabolic disorders and rarer types of genetic abnormalities.

Fig.5.6   The frequency of ovulation in normal women may vary considerably. This is indicated by the density of shadowing in the band below the figure. 'Normal' ovulation includes the whole spectrum.

a. *Spinnbarkheit.* The effect of rising oestrogen levels to the ovulatory peak is to thin out cervical mucus. At the time of ovulation a drop of mucus can be placed on a microscope slide, a second slide placed on top of it and the two slides then separated. Well-oestrogenized mucus will form a thread of 7–8 cm before breaking. After ovulation the effect of progesterone reduces the length of the thread to a centimetre or two.

b. *Ferning.* On the same principle well-oestrogenized cervical mucus, when allowed to dry on a slide and examined under the microscope shows a typical 'fern leaf' pattern. This also disappears after ovulation due to the effect of progesterone.

5. *Visualization of the corpus luteum.* Visualization of the corpus luteum by laparoscopy or laparotomy is good evidence for ovulation having occurred.

6. *Endometrial biopsy.* Histological examination of the endometrium will show secretory changes in the second half of the cycle if ovulation has occurred.

Failure of ovulation may present conventionally as primary or secondary amenorrhoea. Although this is the conventional classification it may, unless used with care, be confusing because 'primary' and 'secondary' are terms used with a different connotation in endocrinology. Furthermore they may not be clearly differentiated clinically. Despite these shortcomings this classification is employed as it is still the one of choice in the majority of textbooks. Only a selected few of the possible causes of amenorrhoea (see Fig. 5.6) can be considered in this book. Other causes, such as general metabolic disorders (e.g. diabetes mellitus), chronic infection (e.g. tuberculosis), and rare types of genetic abnormalities are not discussed. Frequently the reason that medical opinion is sought is a failure to conceive. Polycystic ovarian disease (Stein–Leventhal syndrome), although usually presenting as oligomenorrhoea is for convenience considered in this section. In addition the poor luteal phase syndrome is included, since, although ovulation does in fact occur, successful implantation is not common in this condition and it can be considered as a 'failure of ovulation'.

Although amenorrhoea has been separated into primary and secondary, in practice it may be difficult to differentiate between them in the young.

1. Primary amenorrhoea

The onset of menarche, which can vary, is controlled by the hypothalamic–adenohypophysial axis. The majority of girls in this country have their first period between the ages of 10 and 16 and 50 per cent will be menstruating by the age of 13. The age of onset of the menarche has been falling over the past 100 years but is now thought to be flattening out. The mean is usually said to be $13 \cdot 1 \pm 1$ year.

It is reasonable to delay investigating primary amenorrhoea until the age of 17 years, unless secondary sex characters have developed (i.e. there is a disparity between physical development and the onset of menstruation) or there are other physical signs or symptoms which suggest chromosomal or hormonal abnormalities.

CAUSES:

(a) Cryptomenorrhea. This term means hidden menstruation and is not truly amenorrhoea, as the uterus sheds its endometrium. The menstrual loss is unable to escape due to a transverse septum in the vagina or complete vaginal atresia. The diagnosis is made from a history of cyclical lower abdominal pain with 'menstrual symptoms'. A transverse septum is treated simply by a cruciate incision which allows free drainage. The complete absence of a vagina is a much more difficult problem and plastic surgery is necessary in order to 'construct' one. In addition a laparotomy is performed and if a uterus is present, this is removed. Occasionally the only defect is a failure to connect the uterus and vagina when once again plastic surgery is employed to form a connecting channel.

(b) Delayed menarche. Primary amenorrhoea may prove to be an idiopathic delay in the onset of menstruation. This diagnosis can only be made after all other causes have been excluded. It is a retrospective diagnosis, when eventually menstruation occurs.

(c) Chromosomal. Chromosomal abnormalities are found in one-third of girls with primary amenorrhoea at the age of 18. A chromosomal analysis is therefore an essential investigation. The commonest abnormality is Turner's syndrome (XO chromosomes); the other features of Turner's syndrome (short stature, web neck, coarctation of the aorta) make it likely that the diagnosis will have been made before primary amenorrhoea becomes the significant complaint. However, there may be a few or none of the other clinical features in a patient with Turner's syndrome who has a genetic mosaic (i.e. not all tissues have XO chromosomes). Patients with Turner's syndrome have streak ovaries and do not ovulate. They have poorly developed secondary sex characteristics due to the low level of oestrogens. Menstruation, growth in stature, and development of secondary sex characteristics can be stimulated by oestrogen therapy. After a few months it is usually necessary to add a progestagen in order to achieve full feminization and to reduce the risk of endometrial carcinoma.

(d) Endocrine causes. The main endocrine disorders responsible for primary amenorrhoea are disorders of the adrenal cortex or of the hypothalamic–adenohypophysial axis. It is possible for a patient with congenital adrenal hyperplasia (Chapter 4) to present with primary amenorrhoea. There will be accompanying signs of masculinization. Disturbances of the hypothalamic–adenohypophysial axis such as dwarfism and the Lawrence–Moon–Biedl syndrome† will be associated with amenorrhoea, but usually the conditions have been identified before the age of expected onset of the menarche. Such girls will have associated sexual infantilism.

Patients with hypogonadotrophic eunuchoidism have low levels of plasma FSH and LH and the ovaries will respond to stimulation with exogenous gonadotrophins, unlike patients with true gonadal agenesis who have high levels of gonadotrophins and will not respond to stimulation.

---

† A rare syndrome comprising of mental retardation, hypogonadism, retinitis pigmentosa, obesity, and polydactyly.

(e) End-organ abnormalities. Patients in this category are those with testicular feminization. Chromosome analysis reveals an XY karyotype. The testes may be abdominal or inguinal. The testes produce androgens, but the end-organs, the penis and the breasts, are insensitive to them. The condition is familial and may therefore be seen in other members of the family.

(f) Other causes. It should be remembered that many of the causes of secondary amenorrhoea such as panhypopituitarism and the polycystic ovarian syndrome may rarely be responsible also for primary amenorrhoea.

2. Secondary amenorrhoea

CAUSES:

(a) Polycystic ovarian disease. The Stein–Leventhal syndrome, now known as polycystic ovarian disease, was first described in 1935 by Stein and Levanthal. The original syndrome was one of obesity, hirsutism, infertility, and oligomenorrhoea, although obesity is no longer regarded as part of the syndrome. The biochemistry of the disease is still not clearly understood.

The main defect may be of ovarian origin in most cases, but it may be due to an adrenal cortical disorder since the capsular fibrosis seen in polycystic ovaries may also be seen in the ovaries of those patients with Cushing's syndrome. The increased number of Graafian follicles in the polycystic ovary and the general ovarian enlargement suggests an organ which is being overstimulated. The thickened capsule is known to be associated with the presence of high local androgen concentrations. Not surprisingly, therefore, these patients may have raised plasma testosterone, in addition to raised plasma LH levels.

Partial resection or wedge resection of the ovary has been used for many years to improve the polycystic ovarian syndrome, and this may lead to ovulation. However, the syndrome recurs after wedge resection, and clomiphene has replaced surgery as the elective primary treatment.

(b) Premature menopause or primary ovarian failure is **diagnosed** by symptoms of the menopause coupled with low oestrogen and raised plasma FSH and LH levels.

The aetiology is uncertain but it may be due to premature ageing of the ovaries, when viable ova disappear at an earlier than expected age. In auto-immune Addison's disease antibodies are produced against other hormone-secreting cells, namely the thyroid, pancreas, adenohypophysis, and also possibly the ovaries, the latter resulting in ovarian failure. The condition is incurable, but may be treated symptomatically by oestrogen and progesterone replacement.

(c) Any tumour of the hypothalamus or of the adenohypophysis may interfere with ovulation, and thus menstruation, through the resultant interference with normal adenohypophysial hormone secretion. Currently, the neoplastic condition arousing most interest is the so-called microadenoma of the adenohypophysis which is prolactin-secreting, galactorrhoea sometimes being an additional symptom. Measurement of prolactin is now a routine investigation of all patients with a disturbance of ovulation.

(d) 'Poor luteal phase syndrome' is a diagnosis which is made in infertile

patients when a temperature chart shows a luteal phase which is shorter than the normal 13–14 days. The temperature-rise after ovulation may only be maintained for 4–5 days, or the temperature rise may be inconsistent, varying considerably. The plasma progesterone level is also low.

DIAGNOSIS: The age of onset of menstruation, its frequency, and whether there are any abnormal features should be noted. It is usually important to ascertain whether the patient has been taking the contraceptive pill, or whether she has ever been pregnant. As the patient with galactorrhoea may not mention this change, it is essential to ask whether it is present; it may also only occur on compression of the breast. In contrast any noticeable hairiness, no matter how slight, may be referred to as 'marked hairiness' by the patient. There may be other endocrine disorders besides abnormalities of the menstrual cycle, and the history must encompass these possibilities. It is wise to take a full family history as premature menopause may be present in other members of the family. This gynaecological history is not complete and the reader is referred to a larger textbook for a more detailed account.

A general examination is routinely carried out and the body contour is noted (arm span, height and distribution of hair). The breasts should be compressed to ascertain whether milk can be expressed.

INVESTIGATIONS:

1. An X-ray of the pituitary fossa should be obtained.

2. A routine hormonal investigation is undertaken. Plasma FSH, LH, and prolactin estimations are essential. Some clinicians routinely measure T_3, T_4, and thyrotrophin; others only if there is evidence of thyroid disease. If there is any evidence of virilism or hirsutism the plasma testosterone and the urinary 17-oxosteroid concentrations should be estimated. If the disorder is due to polycystic ovaries the plasma testosterone level may be raised.

3. Visual fields should be determined in any patient with a raised plasma prolactin level, or if it is believed that an adenohypophysial tumour may be present.

4. Gynaecography. Air is injected into the peritoneal cavity and a radiograph is taken of the patient tilted in the head-down position. Abnormalities of the pelvic organs may then be visualized.

5. The chromosome pattern of the patient is determined although genetic abnormalities (presence of Barr bodies) are usually associated with primary amenorrhoea.

6. The value of determining ovarian antibodies in patients with premature menopause in the absence of Addison's disease is debatable.

7. A laparoscopy should be performed to allow close inspection of the ovaries from which a biopsy may be taken and tubal patency demonstrated.

8. An endometrial biopsy is of value to 'date' the endometrium and to exclude tuberculosis.

TREATMENT: The treatment of amenorrhoea is generally best considered as that for infertility. The therapy outlined below is designed for those patients with adenohypophysial ovarian dysfunction only. Naturally, before embarking on what may be an expensive and time-consuming course of treatment, it is necessary to establish that the male partner is fertile.

a. *Clomiphene*. This drug increases the secretion of FSH and LH provided that the hypothalamo-adenohypophysial axis is intact. It may also act directly on ovarian steroidogenesis. Clomiphene is given in a dose of 50 mg daily for each course of 7 days, starting at any time. In patients who are infertile but menstruating, therapy is initiated on the third day after bleeding has ceased. Clomiphene therapy may be combined with an injection of human chorionic gonadotrophin (HCG) for its luteinizing action: 5–10 000 IU is given 4–7 days after the last dose of clomiphene, in order to control the time of ovulation more accurately (for example where artificial insemination is employed). If ovulation is not induced by this dose of clomphene, it can be increased up to 250 mg daily for 5 days.

b. Commercial preparations of *FSH and LH* are available for injection. Gonadotrophins stimulate ovulation very successfully, but oestrogen levels need very careful monitoring during treatment to assess the response of the Graafian follicle and to reduce the risk of hyperstimulation and multiple pregnancy. This should be undertaken only by specialists in this field.

c. *LH releasing hormone* is used to stimulate ovulation, but the results at present are disappointing and details are therefore not given.

d. *Bromocriptine* is used if the blood level of prolactin is high (it has been very successful in the suppression of galactorrhoea). The therapy starts with a small initial dose of 2·5 mg at night and gradually increases to 7·5–10 mg depending on the prolactin level. The possible complication of microadenomata in pregnancy has been discussed previously (Chapter 2). This therapy has also been used in those women who wish to ovulate (i.e. menstruate), but do not wish to become pregnant. The contraceptive pill is contraindicated in these circumstances as prolactin secretion may be stimulated. A barrier method of contraception or the intrauterine contraceptive device should be used.

e. The 'poor luteal phase syndrome' requires *HCG* alone. This is given in a dose of 5000 IU 2–3 days later. Clomiphene may also be used in conjunction with HCG. If pregnancy is not desired, and no abnormality is detected, therapy is not required.

Pre-menstrual tension

This term is used to denote a very varying, complex group of symptoms occurring, as its name implies, at some time during the 10 days before a period.

Fluid retention appears to be part of this syndrome and it is now believed that this is due to the continued action of oestrogen in the latter half of the menstrual cycle. However, it must be emphasized that there may be a considerable emotional component in this condition.

CLINICAL FEATURES: The symptoms include a sensation of lower abdominal discomfort, distension, nausea, breast discomfort, and a general 'bloated feeling'. There may be frequency of micturition, change of bowel habit, an increase or decrease in acne, and a darkening of the skin under the eyes. There is often quite severe depression and reduction of libido.

TREATMENT: Treatment includes oral contraceptives which reduces the total oestrogen secreted between the menses. If this does not help, or in those who do not want to go on the 'pill', progesterone or progestogen may be given in the second half of the cycle. Norethisterone 5 mg, a nortestosterone, may be given by mouth from the first day symptoms appear until the onset of menstruation, or as a 400 mg progesterone suppository. In cases of marked fluid retention, diuretics (such as thiazides) are often a valuable addition to therapy.

Metropathia haemorrhagica (cystic glandular hyperplasia)

This is due to the persistence of a Graafian follicle which fails to rupture but continues to produce oestrogen. This leads to a continuing proliferative phase and endometrial hyperplasia.

As long as the follicular cyst continues to produce oestrogen the endometrium is supported, but as the tension in the follicular cyst rises, the oestrogen production falls and the endometrium is shed. Because of the hyperplasia the bleeding is heavy and may be prolonged. With continuing variable oestrogen production the subsequent bleeding pattern is irregular. Endometrial carcinoma must be excluded and the diagnosis established by histological examination of the curettings. The typical hyperplastic and glandular endometrium is observed.

CLINICAL FEATURES: Clinical presentation of this condition is very typical. The patient is usually in her late 30s or early 40s although occasionally it is found in the younger or over-40 age groups. The menstrual cycle is irregular and there may be heavy vaginal bleeding during the menses.

TREATMENT: Either the combined oral contraceptive pill with a high progesterone content is used or norethisterone is given 5 mg daily from days 15–25. Both of these alternatives may regulate the cycle satisfactorily, but, if not, the only alternative is hysterectomy.

Hirsutism

When considering hirsutism, it is necessary to discuss the sites of androgen secretion (apart from the placenta). While it is accepted that the normal ovaries secrete testosterone, androstenedione and dehydroepiandrosterone, the quantities secreted are insufficient to induce hirsutism. The adrenal cortex is the main source of androgens in the female. However, in pathological states excess androgen secretion inducing hirsutism may be of ovarian as well as adrenal origin. Hence hirsutism may be conveniently considered in this section.

CAUSES: The causes of hirsutism can be divided into the following categories:

1. *Ovarian:*
    i. polycystic ovaries
    ii. ovarian tumours

2. *Adrenal:*
   i. tumours
   ii. hyperplasia $\Big\}$ (see Chapter 4)

3. *Idiopathic*

(a) *Ovarian causes.*
   i. Polycystic ovaries. The typical clinical features of patients with polycystic ovaries (PCO) are infertility, oligomenorrhoea, varying degrees of hirsutism, and obesity. Most patients with PCO have raised levels of testosterone and androstenedione. If the daily production rate of testosterone and androstenedione is measured in patients with PCO these are always found to be raised above the normal female level. The degree of hirsutism bears a close relationship to the level of androgen production.

   Although the precise role of the adrenal gland in this syndrome is uncertain, the results of adrenal and ovarian stimulation and suppression tests indicate that the adrenals in some patients with PCO make a significant contribution to the androgen levels.

   ii. Ovarian tumours: Adrenal and ovarian tumours are the commonest cause of extreme hirsutism and virilism, and differentiation between them is difficult. Generally, if the excess androgens are not reduced with the dexamethasone suppression test the cause is a tumour. Stimulation with corticotrophin (ACTH) is ineffective in patients with ovarian tumours. The diagnosis is confirmed by selective catheterization of the ovarian and adrenal veins. The determination of androgen levels in these venous samples is then used to determine the site of production of the excess hormone.

(b) *Idiopathic hirsutism.* The term 'idiopathic hirsutism' includes those women who are hirsute, but do not have demonstrable adrenal or ovarian pathology. The mean concentrations of the plasma androgens are raised above the normal levels, and these are usually, but not invariably, related to the degree of hirsutism. It is probable that the source of the additional androgens is adrenal. Nevertheless, the possibility remains that the ovary may be the source or that both adrenals and ovaries may be contributing to the increased androgen levels. There remains the as yet, still unexplained observation that apparently normal ovaries may produce excessive androgens and induce hirsutism and even some degree of virilism.

   Another possible explanation of idiopathic hirsutism is increased sensitivity of hair follicles to normal levels of circulating androgen. Eastern women are known to have appreciably less body hair than occidental women with the same levels of androgens. Conversely women from around the Mediterranean basin are appreciably more hirsute than other Europeans. The most extreme example of altered androgen sensitivity is the testicular feminization syndrome where there are high levels of testosterone, but a definite feminine hair growth and distribution.

Hormone-secreting ovarian tumours

These rare conditions are only briefly considered.

1. Oestrogen-secreting tumours

The granulosa and theca cells are responsible for oestrogen secretion and it is the rare tumours of these ovarian cells which produce significant amounts of oestrogen. Many other ovarian tumours may produce small amounts of oestrogens.

Granulosa and theca cell tumours occur most frequently after the menopause, although they may occur earlier. The tumours are solid and small. They may be so small as to be impalpable on vaginal examination even in the slimmest of patients.

The symptoms are related to an increased oestrogen production and include post-menopausal bleeding, an increase in libido, an increase in vaginal moisture, and a general feeling of youthfulness. The endometrium becomes hyperplastic due to unopposed oestrogen action and there may occasionally be an associated endometrial carcinoma.

It is stated that less than one-half of these tumours are malignant and metastases and recurrences are relatively rare. Treatment is nevertheless the removal of both ovaries and uterus. Many gynaecologists also recommend postoperative external irradiation.

2. Androgen-secreting tumours

The arrhenoblastoma and the disgerminoma are the two commonest virilizing ovarian tumours. They tend to arise in younger age groups, certainly premenopausally.

The symptoms produced are those of increasing androgen production: hirsutism, amenorrhoea, clitoral hypertrophy, acne, and voice changes (Chapter 4).

The diagnosis cannot be established without a laparoscopy or laparotomy. Whether to excise one ovary or both and whether to remove the uterus are difficult decisions which will depend on the age of the patient and the degree of malignancy as determined by histological examination.

3. Human chorionic gonadotrophin secreting tumours

Some malignant ovarian cysts produce HCG. This is particularly relevant clinically in a young girl with an ovarian cyst and amenorrhoea. With a positive pregnancy test one can be misled into assuming the mass to be the pregnant uterus rather than a malignant cyst.

The menopause

By definition menopause is the stage in the woman's life when menstruation ceases. However, the systemic changes associated with the menopause may occur before, or months after cessation of menstruation and thus the menopause is the term used to embrace their occurrence. The menopause may be associated with the belief that there is a loss of physical attraction and of 'unwantedness'. At the same time the children are at an age when they are seeking their own self-expression outside the home, and the woman feels that she has lost her 'motherhood'. Whether these factors are divorced from other psychological changes such as depression, irritability, and lassitude is uncertain. Furthermore, it is important to appreciate that the social environment of many women is such that their role in life is regarded as mainly to produce children and to perform household duties; an attitude which still persists in this country even in the late 1970s. The woman's reaction to the menopause may in addition be influenced by religious factors. These psychological effects and the social background have to be considered when assessing the significance of the hormonal changes which may be wholly or in part responsible for the mental effects. It is this uncertainty of the cause of the psychological disturbances and the effect these may have on the response of the patient to the 'organic changes' which accentuates the problems of justifying hormonal replacement therapy. It must be emphasized that many women are not troubled by the menopause. It has been observed that women who are least troubled by the menopause are those with a stable marriage and who have had children.

A low oestradiol level is responsible for the atrophy of the breasts, labia, uterus, and vaginal epithelium; the associated dryness of the vagina renders this organ more susceptible to infection. The low level of the hormone may contribute to uterine prolapse and susceptibility to bladder infections. It has been claimed that the fall of oestrogen levels is responsible for a rise in the plasma cholesterol concentration, which may be related to an increased incidence of cardiovascular disease. The other symptoms of the menopause appear to be more associated with the rise in the adenohypophysial hormones than a fall in gonadal hormones. These symptoms include vasomotor flushes and sweating; emotional instability, obesity, and hirsutism. The thinning of the skin and loss of pubic hair may be associated with ovarian degeneration and possible loss of androgen secretion. It has been claimed that a low blood oestradiol concentration is associated with a reduction of libido, but it is exceedingly difficult to separate this change from associated emotional factors.

Senile osteoporosis is an organic change which is closely associated with a long period of low oestradiol levels such as occurs in postmenopausal women.

TREATMENT: The problem of therapy for the menopause is perplexing. Whether hormone replacement therapy should be used to maintain 'youthfulness' is debatable. It is generally agreed that therapy is justified if the symptoms are causing distress. This therapy is often necessary in premature menopause, either occurring naturally or induced by obliteration of the ovaries by radiotherapy or surgery.

Oestrogens may be replaced orally, by injection, or by implantation of an oestrogen pellet. The benefits of oestrogen replacement are undoubted when severe menopausal symptoms are due to oestrogen deficiency; the benefits are more variable where there is marked emotional overlay. If the major problem is vaginal, an oestrogen cream is of value.

The action of hormonal contraceptives

1. The combined oestrogen–progestogen pill

Most combined pills contain 30 or 50 μg of an oestrogen with varying amounts of progestogen. Progesterone itself is not adequately absorbed from the upper gastrointestinal tract and this means that another, synthetic progestogen has to be used.

The effect of the combined pill is to inhibit ovulation. This effect is achieved by depressing the secretion of gonadotrophin-releasing hormone by the hypothalamus, thus preventing the release of LH. It may also inhibit the release of the adenohypophysial gonadotrophin by a direct effect rather than by inhibiting its synthesis. FSH and LH are present in only basal amounts in the patient on the pill and the mid-cycle peak of LH is abolished.

Consequent upon this mechanism there are changes in the ovaries (no mature Graafian follicles and no corpora lutea) and in the endometrium which may become atrophic because it can never undergo adequate proliferation. The continuous cyclical administration of the combined pill usually results in immature follicles and even if a follicle should mature there is no sudden surge of LH to induce ovulation. Also the cervical mucus remains thick and viscous due to the influence of progesterone. The motility of the Fallopian tubes is also suppressed.

2. Progestogen-only pills

The progestogen-only contraceptives, whether given by injection or by mouth act in the following ways:

1. All progestogens have an inhibitory effect on ovulation.
2. Meiosis is interfered with.
3. The cervical mucus is thick and impenetrable.
4. Tubular motility is changed and altered such that fertilization becomes impossible.
5. Should ovulation take place the function of the corpus luteum is altered and progesterone levels in the second half of the cycle are relatively low.
6. The endometrial glands become inactive and prevent implantation, even if fertilization occurs.

Despite these multiple actions, which appear impregnable, pregnancy nevertheless may occur. Furthermore, bleeding is often irregular.

DISORDERS OF THE MALE OR FEMALE

Precocious puberty

The age of onset of puberty is influenced by race, nutrition, and genetic constitution. It is currently believed that some particular body weight determines the onset of puberty. The mean age of the menarche is about 13·1 years, while in the male the testicles begin to enlarge at about 12 years; the standard deviation of both means is approximately 1 year. When maturation of adenohypophysial-gonadal function occurs at a premature age (i.e. before 8 years in girls and 10 years in boys), reference is made to true precocious sexual puberty, which is a very rare condition. Pseudoprecocious puberty is considered as the condition which arises when there is an inappropriately high level of sex hormones due to some disorder of the gonads or adrenal cortex. In the female it is important to distinguish two particular conditions from precocious puberty. First, when the breast develops at an early age without any other sexual development and secondly when the only premature development is axillary and pubic hair (either one or the other may be present). These are accepted as deviations from the normal.

No cause can be discovered in the majority of females with precocious sexual development, but when the cause is due to pathological disorders the majority have ovarian diseases. In contrast, pathological disorders are more commonly the cause of this condition in boys; the aetiology in about 50 per cent is equally divided between intracranial and adrenal diseases; occasionally the fault is testicular, but usually the source is unknown.

Before considering true and pseudoprecocious sexual development it is useful to consider some important aspects involved in their differentiation. The basic difference between true and pseudoprecocious puberty is that in the former condition mature gametes are present in the gonads which are fully developed (e.g. testicles of adult size). Cyclic menstruation in the female has been described in the pseudo variety and therefore the presence or absence of menstrual cycles cannot be used as a diagnostic differentiation.

True sexual precocity

CAUSES:

(a) Disorders of the central nervous system. Usually the pathological changes are found in the hypothalamic region posterior to the median eminence, but when a hamartoma (normal tissue in an ectopic site) is the cause this tumour may be anterior to this structure. As hamartomata are not invariably associated with precocity it has been suggested that they only produce this effect when there are neuronal connections between the tumour and the brain. Brain tumours (gliomata, astrocytomata) in the region of the third ventricle and even craniopharyngiomas may also induce precocity. There has always been an interest in tumours of the pineal gland, but it seems likely that these tumours, when they induce sexual precocity, are teratomata (Plate 5.1). The relationship between the pineal gland and the development of puberty in man is still undecided. It would appear that in those patients with pinealomata (not teratomata) and sexual precocity the changes are secondary, induced by pressure effects on the hypothalamus.

(b) Idiopathic. The diagnosis is based on the absence of any definite disorders of the central nervous system, although a large number of these patients have abnormal EEG patterns and may have epilepsy (Plate 5.2). Occasionally the condition is familial in which case it is usually the males that are affected.

(c) Hypothyroidism. A rare, but interesting association occurs between hypothyroidism and precocious sexual puberty, but interest in the condition really stems from the fact that replacement with thyroxine restores normality.

CLINICAL FEATURES: It is unusual to see patients less than 4 years old, although medical literature contains discussions of such children. Sexual development is then obviously advanced as is bone age revealed by radiography except in patients with hypothyroidism. Growth as expected is rapid at first, but fusion of the epiphyses occurs early and the final result is a patient of short stature. Curiously, dentition is not advanced.

In girls some mental retardation may be present, while in boys it is claimed

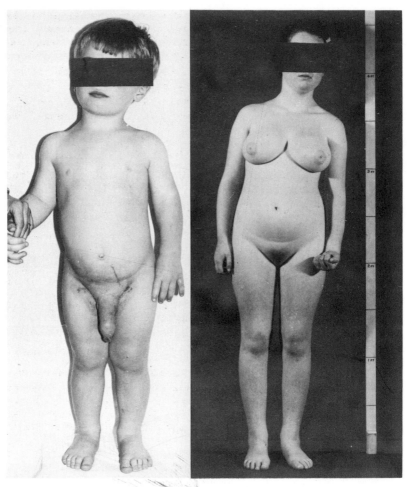

Plate 5.1   A boy aged 4 with true precocious puberty due to a teratoma. The testes are undescended but the penis is of adult proportions.

Plate 5.2   A girl aged 7 with true precocious puberty. No cause was found although the patient was fully investigated. A laparotomy revealed no abnormalities. An EEG showed a typical epileptiform pattern.

that the IQ is raised. Girls, even though physically mature, are not psychologically adapted to cope with their precocity; however, boys may have some psychological sex drive, but this is usually in the form of sexual fantasies.

Family history may reveal that relatives have also had precocious sexual development. Careful enquiries should be made about any episodes of unconsciousness, fits, etc. in the patient. Physical examination reveals that the external genitalia are of adult proportions. In females it may be wise to have a full pelvic examination under an anaesthetic, so that a careful palpation of the genital tract can be made to determine whether there is any ovarian enlargement. In addition, a full medical examination is necessary in order to determine if there are any associated changes such as abnormal pigmentation of the skin.

INVESTIGATIONS: Although the blood gonadotrophins are not raised above normal adult levels they are high with respect to the chronological age. Similarly the plasma levels of gonadal hormones are comparatively raised. These estimations provide confirmatory evidence if required.

The differential diagnosis of true from pseudoprecocity in the male is the finding of an adult sperm-count; occasionally testicular biopsy may be of value.

In females the pseudo type is usually due to a granulosa cell tumour which is frequently palpable. The gonadotrophic hormone blood-levels are low, but normal for age.

In order to differentiate the idiopathic variety from that due to neurological changes, it is necessary to carry out a full neurological investigation including skull X-ray arteriography or air encephalogram. An EMI brain scanner will probably replace these invasive techniques.

TREATMENT: If a cranial tumour is present, it is removed. The treatment of hypothyroidism has been considered in chapter 6. The idiopathic variety is difficult to treat but psychological therapy may result in some improvement. The value of medroxyprogesterone in females and cyproterone acetate in the male has yet to be evaluated in this condition.

Pseudo-precocious puberty

CAUSES: The causes of pseudoprecocious puberty are considered below:

(a) Tumours of the ovary. The usual tumour which induces pseudo precocity is a granulosa cell tumour. Very occasionally the tumour is a teratoma theca cell tumour or an arrhenoblastoma. Another type of teratoma, chorionepithelioma, may develop in the ovary and can induce precocity.

(b) Tumours of the testes. The tumour may be a seminoma, teratoma, or chorionepithelioma.

(c) Adrenal tumours. Carcinoma of the adrenals may produce androgens which in young boys can produce precocious puberty. It is rarely a cause of precocity in females. The condition must be distinguished from congenital adrenal hyperplasia (see Chapter 4).

(d) Fibrous dysplasia (Albright's syndrome). This is a rare cause of precocity which is usually classified as the pseudo variety. There is a characteristic brownish pigmentation of the skin (see Plate 5.3).

(e) Factitious. There have been reports of female children accidentally ingesting large quantities of oestrogens which induce precocity. In boys iatrogenic precocity has been induced by the overenthusiastic administration of gonadotrophins for cryptorchidism.

CLINICAL FEATURES: Examination follows the same pattern as that described for true precocity, and changes such as patchy pigmentation of the skin may be

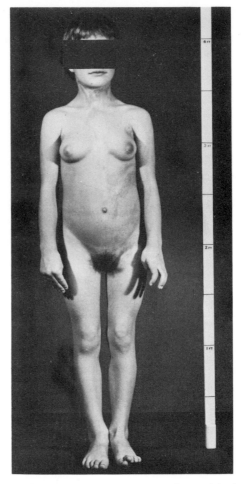

Plate 5.3   A girl aged 5 with Albright's syndrome. Note the characteristic pigmentation especially on the left side of the trunk and around the neck.

observed in the general examination (Albright's syndrome). Any degree of virilism in females indicates that the underlying pathology is usually of adrenal cortical and only rarely of ovarian origin (arrhenoblastoma). While the female may have some type of cyclical bleeding, both the male and the female are infertile in this condition.

INVESTIGATIONS: In chorionephithelioma the gonadotrophins in the blood and urine are raised; furthermore, the pregnancy test is positive in females.

With the other causes the trophic hormones are low (i.e. normal for age) but the levels of gonadal hormones are relatively high for age. In a granulosa cell tumour the oestrogen level may even exceed that seen in an adult woman.

TREATMENT: This usually requires appropriate surgical treatment and for details the reader should consult more specialized reference books.

6 The thyroid gland

PHYSIOLOGY

The thyroid gland secretes the metabolic hormones thyroxine (tetraiodothyronine) and triiodothyronine, which regulate the oxygen consumption of the majority of cells; in the normal state the quantities secreted by the gland ensure that the cellular metabolism is optimal. The concentration of the metabolic hormones in the blood is controlled by an adenohypophysial hormone, thyrotrophin (thyroid-stimulating hormone, TSH).

Another thyroidal hormone, calcitonin, is secreted from parafollicular cells (C cells) and this hormone is concerned with calcium metabolism. Detailed consideration of calcitonin is given in Chapter 7.

Anatomy, histology, and development

The thyroid develops as a diverticulum in the middle of the floor of the primitive endodermal pharynx. The diverticulum becomes bi-lobed, and is attached by the thyroglossal duct to the floor of the pharynx as the foramen caecum where the anterior two-thirds and the posterior one-third of the developing tongue meet. Normally this duct disappears. Part of the fourth pharyngeal endodermal pouch and the ultimobranchial body from the fifth pouch are incorporated into the developing thyroid, and it is thought that the parafollicular cells arise from them.

The gland is composed of follicles which consist of an outer layer of follicular cells resting on a basement membrane and enclosing an amorphous material called colloid. These follicles are embedded in stromal tissue which contains blood-vessels and autonomic nerve fibres. Enhanced activity of the gland is revealed by a decrease in the quantity of colloid with the subsequent reduction of follicular volume, while the lining cells become columnar and may even proliferate into the colloid. Enlargement of the follicle due to accumulation of colloid with a flattening of the follicular cells occurs in decreased activity.

Increased magnification shows that there are gaps between the endothelial cells of the capillaries. The follicular cell cytoplasm has a microtubular network and from the apices of these follicular cells there are microvilli containing canuliculi which project into the colloid. These cells in common with those of many other endocrine glands have a prominent endoplasmic reticulum.

Metabolic hormones (thyroxine and triiodothyronine)

Synthesis, storage, and release

The important element involved in the synthesis of the two metabolic hormones of the thyroid gland is iodine, which is normally ingested in the form of iodides. The follicular cells concentrate iodides by means of an active pump mechanism to some 25–50 times the normal plasma levels. The activity of this 'iodide pump' is controlled by thyrotrophin (TSH) from the adenohypophysis. Once inside the cell, iodide is rapidly oxidized to the more reactive iodine by a peroxidase enzyme. The iodine then becomes incorporated into tyrosine amino-acid groups which form part of a thyroidal protein called thyroglobulin (mol. wt about 660 000), also synthesized within the follicular cells before being secreted into the colloid. It is generally considered that the synthesis of the two hormones triiodothyronine and tetraiodothyronine (T_3 and T_4) results from an internal coupling reaction between mono- and di-iodotyrosyl groups on the thyroglobulin which necessitates structural changes in the molecule. The synthesis of T_3 and T_4 on the thyroglobulin molecule occurs mainly at the follicular cell–colloid interface, and also within the colloid. The thyroglobulin is present in the highest concentrations within the colloid, where it is stored. The follicular cells engulf globules of colloid by endocytosis, and this process, together with the subsequent breakdown of the thyroglobulin molecules by lysosomal proteases, is again under the influence of TSH. (Recent evidence suggests that the intracellular microtubular network in the follicular cells may also be involved in the uptake of thyroglobulin.) Any mono- and di-iodotyrosine molecules (T_1 and T_2) released into the follicular cell cytoplasm are broken down to iodide and tyrosyl groups which can then be re-utilized. The two hormones T_3 and T_4 are released into the blood by diffusion (see Fig. 6.1).

In the blood, the two hormones are transported mostly bound to certain plasma proteins; T_4 is mainly bound to thyroxine-binding globulin (TBG), and in part to thyroxine-binding prealbumin, and to albumin. The other hormone (T_3) is less avidly bound, and principally to the prealbumin and albumin. The active components of both blood-borne hormones are the unbound (free) fractions, which consist of approximately 0·024 per cent of the total T_4 and 0·5 per cent of the total T_3. This relatively small difference between the active fractions of the two hormones may account for their differing potencies. Furthermore, the delay of action (latency) for T_3 and T_4 is about 12 h and 72 h respectively, while their peak effects occur within 1–2 days for T_3 and after 7–9 days for T_4.

Actions

The hormones have many actions, but the primary one is a calorigenic (increased oxygen consumption) effect on many tissues, possibly by decreasing the efficiency of intracellular oxidative phosphorylation. However there are some tissues, for example the brain, retinae, testes, lungs, and spleen which do not appear to be affected by this action of the hormones. In mammals the hormones also influence growth and maturation and aid in the regulation of lipid metabolism. Other actions can be accounted for by increased sensitivity of the β-receptors to catecholamines, e.g. adrenalin.

The increased oxygen consumption which is observed following T_4 administration results in an increased basal metabolic rate. This calorigenic effect may partly follow the stimulation of protein synthesis which is induced by the thyroidal metabolic hormones. This anabolic response appears to be dependent upon the metabolic state of the animal and the dose of hormone adminis-

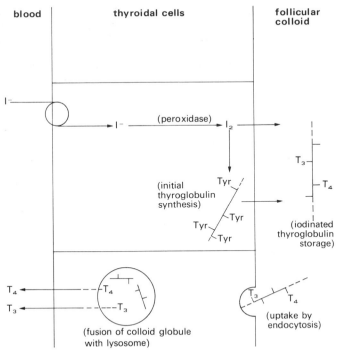

Fig.6.1   The principal stages involved in the synthesis and release of tri-iodothyronine and thyroxine (T_3 and T_4) from the thyroid gland. Some iodination of thyroglobulin occurs within the cells.

tered. Normal blood-levels of thyroid hormones enhance protein anabolism and are thus essential for growth. An excess of the hormones however induces a net increase in protein catabolism which retards physical growth. A deficiency (impaired protein anabolism) or an excess (enhanced protein catabolism) of T_4 will therefore retard physical development.

Thyroid hormones influence carbohydrate metabolism in many ways; they generally stimulate cellular metabolism by enhancing the effects of other hormones such as the catecholamines, and by certain direct effects of their own. For example, glycogenolysis induced by adrenalin is enhanced by thyroid hormones possibly by increasing the sensitivity of the adenyl cyclase–cyclic AMP system. In addition thyroid hormones potentiate the effects of insulin on increasing glucose uptake in adipose tissue and in muscle, and also potentiate insulin-induced glycogen synthesis. One direct effect of thyroid hormones is to stimulate the rate of intestinal glucose absorption.

Thyroid hormones stimulate the synthesis, the mobilization, and the degradation of lipids, with the degradation effect being the more prominent. Lipolysis in adipose tissue is stimulated both by a direct effect of T_3 and T_4 on the adenyl cyclase–cyclic AMP system and by sensitizing the tissue to other lipolytic agents such as catecholamines and glucagon. The increased lipolysis results in increased quantities of these substrates entering the liver which in turn leads to increased hepatic synthesis of triglycerides. However the degradation of lipids is increased to a greater extent than their synthesis so that in the presence of excess thyroid hormones there is a net decrease in the stores of fats and usually a fall in concentration of circulating plasma lipids (e.g. triglycerides, cholesterol, phospholipids). There may be an increase in the plasma concentrations of cholesterol and other lipids when thyroid hormone levels are lowered.

As a result of the increased basal metabolic rate induced by the thyroidal hormones, there is necessarily an increased need for coenzymes, and therefore for the vitamins from which many are derived. However the thyroidal hormones are themselves necessary for various conversions of vitamins to coenzymes, and also for the metabolism of some of the vitamins. For example, the hepatic conversion of carotenes to vitamin A is dependent on the actions of T_3 and T_4. In hypothyroidism the plasma carotene level can increase so much that the skin may develop a yellowish tinge, and symptoms of vitamin A deficiency may be present.

Thyroid hormones are essential for the normal development of the central nervous system, so that insufficiency or lack at birth results in poor development of cellular processes, hypoplasia of cortical neurones, and retarded myelination of nerve fibres. If the deficiency is not corrected within weeks of birth irreversible damage occurs. In the adult, hypothyroidism is characterized by poor mentation, lack of memory, and poor initiative. Psychological changes may often occur, and these are usually depression or paranoia. The effects of thyroidal hormones on cortical arousal are believed to be due, at least partly, to a potentiation of the effects of catecholamines.

Control of release

It is now accepted that the plasma level of thyrotrophin (TSH) controls the rates of synthesis and secretion of T_4 and T_3. The plasma concentration of the active (free) hormones in turn plays a major role in controlling the rate of TSH secretion such that an increase in active T_4 or T_3 inhibits, and a decrease stimulates, the release of TSH. This inverse relationship by negative feedback ensures that under normal conditions the levels of the hormones are maintained within relatively narrow limits. The release of TSH is primarily under the control of a hypothalamic releasing hormone TRH (see Chapter 2), and there is evidence to suggest that the negative feedback by T_4 and T_3 occurs at two levels: the adenohypophysis and the hypothalamus. In addition the rate of secretion of TSH is influenced by various emotional factors, and possibly by exposure to cold, through their effect on the hypothalamus. The actions of TSH include (1) the stimulation of the iodide pump in the cell membranes; (2) stimulation of thyroglobulin synthesis; (3) stimulation of colloidal uptake by the follicular cells; and (4) increased rate of proteolysis of thyroglobulin. In addition it induces an increase in size and number of the thyroidal follicular cells. Prolonged TSH stimulation leads to increased vascularity of the gland and, eventually to hypertrophy. Any enlargement of the thyroid is called a goitre.

CLINICAL DISORDERS

Some authorities claim that thyroid malfunction is even more common than diabetes mellitus. There is a prevalence of thyroid malfunction in females. The clinical picture is due to over- or under-activity of the gland. Hyperthyroidism must always be considered in any patient who is anxious, flushed, sweaty, and losing weight. The presenting symptom may be irritability, which is frequently complained of by the spouse! In middle age the disease can present as atrial fibrillation with or without heart failure. Hypothyroidism (myxoedema) may develop so insidiously that neither the patient nor the immediate family appreciate the changes. These may include an increase in weight, although changes of weight are not invariable in either the hypo- or the hyperthyroid patient. Of clinical interest is the observation that following replacement therapy the patient loses the placidity and pleasantness which are common characteristics of myxoedema. It must be emphasized that many elderly patients may have the typical appearance of myxoedema without having the disease. One particular group of patients could be considered separately on clinical grounds because their condition changes from the hyper- to the hypothyroid state.

Thyrotoxicosis is considered as one condition, although it is appreciated that clinically it is sometimes divided into two categories: thyrotoxicosis in the young associated with typical eye changes and with diffuse enlargement of the thyroid (Graves' disease), and thyrotoxicosis, occurring more commonly in an older age group, with nodular enlargement of the thyroid but no eye changes. Certain additional aspects of the malfunction are mentioned in this chapter.

The aetiologies of hyperthyroidism and hypothyroidism are of interest as autoimmune factors have been implicated; now, many would regard these as being mainly responsible for the two disorders, after iodine deficiency has been excluded.

Thyroid hormone disorders

Excess

Thyrotoxicosis (hyperthyroidism)

The presence of excess circulating thyroid hormone, whether T_4, T_3 or both, is called thyrotoxicosis (the clinical term) or hyperthyroidism. Apart from the occasional case due to excess ingestion of thyroxine 'thyrotoxicosis factitia' hyperthyroidism is nearly always due to disease of the thyroid gland itself. Hyperthyroidism induced by ectopic secretion of TSH is exceedingly rare.

AETIOLOGY: Almost all non-ocular symptoms and signs in thyrotoxicosis are dependent on excess circulating levels of T_4 and T_3. Autoimmune antibodies can be demonstrated in the sera of almost all patients with hyperthyroidism complicated by ophthalmopathy (Graves' disease). 'Long-acting thyroid stimulating antibody', LATS (peak action at about 24 h compared with TSH at about 3 h), has been known and investigated for many years, but its role in the mechanism of hyperthyroidism remains dubious, as it can be demonstrated in only approximately 50 per cent of patients. It is one of a group of IgG antibodies the most important of which, now shown to be present in over 90 per cent of patients with Graves' disease, is 'human specific thyroid stimulating antibody' (HTS).

Stimulation of the target gland by autoantibodies (e.g. by HTS on the thyroid gland), is a most unusual manifestation of antibodies, which more commonly have a destructive potential. When thyroid antibodies of any type are present in the serum there is also a higher incidence of other organ-specific autoantibodies such as those for gastric parietal cells and adrenal cortical cells, though they are not necessarily associated with disease. Similarly, thyroid antibodies occur in the absence of clinical thyroid disease in some 15 per cent of the normal British population.

The current concept of the cause of thyrotoxicosis is that an autoimmune disorder, the underlying nature of which is still not known, results in the production of HTS. Under these circumstances physiological control of the thyroid gland would no longer operate normally.

The eye signs of Graves' disease may possibly result from the presence of a factor (which may or may not be an antibody) termed exophthalmos-producing substance (EPS). Its structure and character must be established before the role of such a substance is accepted.

The precipitating factors in most other forms of hyperthyroidism are not known. One exception is the Jod–Basedow phenomenon in which hyper-thyroidism is induced by the administration of iodine to a patient with a hyperplastic thyroid gland secondary to iodine deficiency.

CLINICAL FEATURES: Signs and symptoms of the hyperthyroid state result from the generalized increase in basal metabolic rate and from the specific effects of the hormone on some organs. Fatigue, irritability, or agitation, weight loss despite voracious appetite, excessive sweating with heat into-lerance, and palpitations are common. The hair is usually fine and the nails thin and brittle. Menstrual irregularities, usually oligo- or amenorrhoea, are com-mon. Eye complaints such as double or blurred vision, a 'burning sensation', and rarely decreased visual acuity may occur. Less commonly there may be dyspnoea and diarrhoea. Some of these symptoms are frequently found in anxiety states and the differential diagnosis cannot always be made clinically.

On examination the patient fidgets and appears anxious; the eyes may stare and protrude. Usually there is persistent tachycardia, fine tremor, and abnor-mal sweating which is frequently apparent in the hands which are hot and sweaty.

Careful examination of the eyes and the thyroid gland is essential. Detect-able ocular abnormalities are considerably more common than actual eye complaints. Eyelid retraction, allowing the sclera to be seen above the limbus of the cornea (Plates 6.1 and 6.2), swelling of the eyelids, infection of the conjuctivae, lid-lag, and proptosis (forward protrusion of the eyeball) with or without ocular palsy may be present; of the latter the commonest defect is a failure of movement of the eyes in an upward and outward direction, some-times with an impaired lateral movement. Defects are often unilateral, and need not be restricted to one muscle.

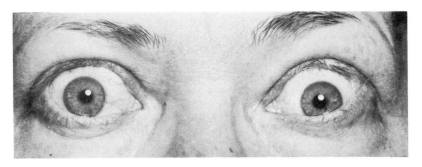

Plate 6.1   The characteristic eyelid retraction in a patient with thyrotoxicosis.

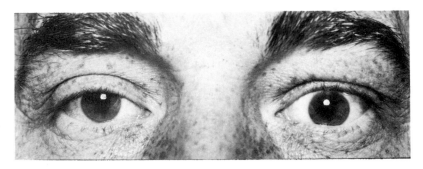

Plate 6.2   Unilateral lid retraction (left eyelid) in a patient with thyrotoxicosis.

The thyroid gland may be palpable in a considerable number of normal people. Therefore on examination it is essential to assess its size and whether it is pathologically enlarged (a goitre). It is important to determine if nodules are present, noting their distribution, and also whether a bruit can be heard over the gland. If there is any suspicion of a retrosternal extension of a goitre (e.g. excessive dyspnoea or wheezing) radiology of the thoracic inlet is much more accurate than the clinical manoeuvres sometimes described.

Important variants described under the two names 'thyrotoxic heart disease' and 'apathetic thyroid disease' must always be considered. In contrast to classical thyrotoxicosis, which usually occurs in patients between 20 and 30 years, these conditions more commonly affect an older age group. Patients with cardiac failure and persistent tachycardia or atrial fibrillation which are often resistant to large doses of digoxin (particularly in the absence of clinically detectable ischaemic heart disease) may be suffering from thyrotoxic heart disease. Other typical clinical signs are commonly absent, although some loss in weight is not infrequent. A similar picture of cardiac failure with weight loss in association with severe apathy, lethargy or depression and with biochemical indices of hyperthyroidism has been termed 'apathetic thyroid disease'.

Pre-tibial myxoedema, thyroid acropachy ('finger clubbing' see p. 122), vitiligo, gynaecomastia, or splenomegaly occur in less than 10 per cent of thyrotoxic patients. Glycosuria with its associated symptoms and impaired glucose tolerance are occasionally the first indication of thyroid disease. Weakness may be due to an underlying thyrotoxic myopathy, which affects the proximal part of the limb, but more commonly it is due to the generalized effect of thyrotoxicosis. Osteoporosis, hypercalcaemia, and hypercalciuria are rarely of clinical significance.

INVESTIGATIONS:

1. Estimation of protein bound iodide (PBI) with its numerous problems is obsolete as circulating thyroid hormones can now be readily measured. Free-T_4 and free-T_3 may prove to be more valuable estimations than the total (bound and free hormone) T_4 and T_3 which are used in most laboratories. The free hormone can either be directly measured or calculated from total levels by a variety of methods (Chapter 12). Most thyrotoxic patients will have a raised free-T_4 and an associated raised free-T_3. Usually no further diagnostic test is required. Increased free-T_3 in the presence of normal free-T_4 ('T_3-toxicosis') is well recognized although infrequent. Raised free-T_3 alone however does not invariably mean that the patient is hyperthyroid, as this may occur, for example, following radio-iodine ablative therapy.

2. Where the diagnosis remains in doubt a thyrotrophin-releasing hormone (TRH) test is helpful. If there is an increased plasma TSH following administration of TRH the subject is not thyrotoxic.

3. Thyroid antibodies (antibodies to thyroid follicular cells or to thyro-globulin) and iodine studies are of little diagnostic importance when thyroid hormones can themselves be measured. Indeed any further necessary investigation relates to treatment rather than to diagnosis and is outlined in the following section.

TREATMENT: Three forms of therapy are available for hyperthyroidism: drug therapy, surgery, and ablative radioiodine.

Drug therapy. Drug therapy is satisfactory for most classic cases in young subjects. The presence of thyroid antibodies in high titre indicates this treatment, as this is a manifestation of extensive lymphoid infiltration of the thyroid which may itself eventually render the patient hypothyroid. Thioureas, usually carbimazole, are commonly used. The half-life is short (6 h) and they are best given three or four times daily. For initial control 40 mg carbimazole daily is usually sufficient, which can later be reduced to a maintenance dose of 15–30 mg. Response is best monitored by clinical evidence of suppression of the toxicosis and repeated TSH estimations for evidence of overtreatment. The most common side-effect of thioureas are skin rashes and agranulocytosis. If skin rashes occur with one preparation of thiourea it may not with another in the same patient. The routine white cell counts are not however helpful in the diagnosis of the blood disorder, since agranulocytosis generally develops within a few days. As a precaution, therefore, patients should be advised to discontinue taking the drug if they develop a sore throat (even though many will not have agranulocytosis).

An alternative group of drugs are the beta-blockers. These relieve the symptoms and improve some of the clinical signs, although they do not affect the basal metabolic rate. They can be of therapeutic value for the rapid relief of symptoms, but their place in long-term management is more debatable.

Whichever medical treatment is used, the aim is to control the disease until it remits in accordance with its natural history. Therapy is usually continued for between 18 and 24 months after which over 50 per cent will be in remission. During therapy the goitre may enlarge, but seldom sufficiently to warrant cessation of treatment; a decrease in the size of the goitre only occurs rarely.

Surgical treatment. Surgical treatment by partial thyroidectomy is employed in the presence of tracheal obstruction. It is also used when relapse occurs after adequate medical treatment, for single autonomous thyroid nodules and occasionally for purely cosmetic reasons. Thyroid scanning is helpful pre-operatively to outline the full extent of thyroid tissue and to demonstrate 'hot' nodules (i.e. nodules having a high uptake of radioactive iodine). Post-operative complications both immediate (bleeding, hypocalcaemia) and subsequent (hypoparathyroidism, recurrent laryngeal nervy palsy, hypothyroidism) may occur. Hypothyroidism is by far the most common complication. Control of the toxic state pre-operatively and careful postoperative supervision are essential to prevent the onset of a thyroid crisis (Chapter 11).

Ablative radio-iodine. Ablative radio-iodine treatment is often the treatment of choice for elderly patients who are less suitable for operation and who are less likely to follow rigid medical regime.

Relapsed thyrotoxicosis may also be treated in this way in younger patients. In this country radio-iodine is not usually given in therapeutic dosage to females who are in the reproductive phase of life. However, evidence now suggests this to be an unnecessary safeguard, provided the patient is not pregnant at the time of treatment. Because the destruction of thyroid tissue may lead to a rapid outpouring of thyroid hormone and precipitation of a thyroid crisis it may be advisable to control the thyroid state by medical means in the more severely affected patients and in the elderly before radio-iodine administration. Two further disadvantages of this therapy are the delay of several months before the treatment is fully effective and the high incidence of hypothyroidism on long-term follow-up. The latter is discovered in over 10 per cent of cases after one year and probably over 50 per cent after 10 years, although it is obviously dependent upon the dose of radio-iodine used.

Deficiency

Hypothyroidism
Deficiency of circulating thyroid hormone may result from primary thyroid disease or secondary to reduced TSH secretion from the adenohypophysis. Myxoedema (primary or secondary) is often used synonymously with hypo-

thyroidism, although some restrict this term only to those patients with pronounced dermal infiltration.

AETIOLOGY: Hypothyroidism may occur due to disorders of thyroid hormone synthesis and the usual cause of this is an iodine deficiency; in some areas there is a low concentration of this element in the drinking water. More commonly autoimmune disease of the thyroid, for example in the late stage of Hashimoto's thyroiditis, or destruction or removal of the gland by surgery or by radioactive iodine treatment give rise to hypothyroidism. The uncommon situation of secondary hypothyroidism (decreased release of TSH) may occur in any condition which gives rise to hypopituitarism.

CLINICAL FEATURES OF THYROIDAL HYPOTHYROIDISM: The majority of patients with hypothyroidism are female and have primary thyroid disease. The presentation of the disease varies in different age groups. The new-born hypothyroid child has a characteristic facies, namely puffiness, low forehead, and an enlarged protuberant tongue; another typical feature is an umbilical hernia. Neurological examination reveals sluggish responses and hypotonia. Untreated the child remains stunted with a low IQ (cretinism) but therapy usually raises the IQ provided it is started as soon as possible; early diagnosis is therefore vital. It is also important to remember that treatment of a pregnant woman with antithyroid drugs can give rise to a goitrous cretinoid infant, in addition to those cases due to iodine deficiency or hereditary defects. Older children may present simply as 'failure to thrive' in the absence of other stigmata of thyroid disease.

Adult patients with myxoedema portray evidence of generalized hypometabolism. Slowness of thought and action, memory impairment, thick dry skin, loss of hair, and intolerance to cold, constipation, and menorrhagia are common. Obesity is less common than is often implied.

On clinical examination the facial appearance is characteristic—a puffy face, especially the lower lids, reddened cheeks, and skin which is often tinged a faint yellow (carotenaemia). The patient, huddled in blankets even on a warm day, slowly replies to questions in a husky voice. There is bradycardia, the skin feels dry and is usually associated with the characteristic subdermal thickening. This infiltration of the skin by mucopolysaccharides occurs initially around the eyes. The body temperature may be lowered. Delayed relaxation of the tendon reflex (the ankle reflex being traditionally used) is a further useful clinical sign. Sometimes in the more severe case there may be effusions into the pleura, pericardium, and peritoneum and the fluid, if obtained, shows the characteristic gold colour due to its high cholesterol content. This typical gross picture of myxoedema is easy to diagnose (see Plates 6.3 and 6.4). However, many patients present with milder degrees of thyroid hypofunction. In these cases, symptoms are often non-specific such as lethargy or hair loss. In addition most physical signs are rarely present. Such cases can only be diagnosed biochemically.

CLINICAL FEATURES OF 'PITUITARY' HYPOTHYROIDISM: Thyrotrophin is usually the third adenohypophysial hormone to be affected in hypopituitarism (preceded by decreased gonadotrophin and somatotrophin). 'Pituitary' (adenohypophysial) or hypothalamic hypothyroidism, while generally milder,

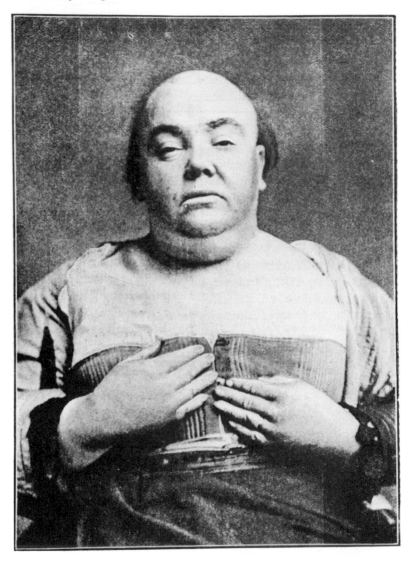

Plate 6.3.(a)   A grocer's wife aged 39 with myxoedema (*Medical Illustrated News* 1889).

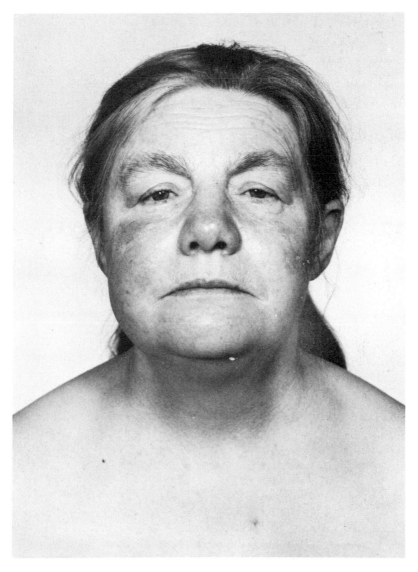

Plate 6.3.(b) A typical myxoedematous female patient aged 47 years.

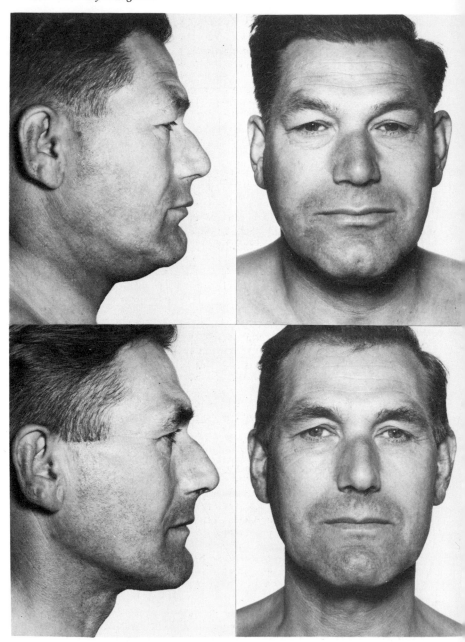

Plate 6.4 *Upper:* Myxoedema in a male patient aged 50 before treatment. *Lower:* the same patient two years after thyroxine therapy. An interesting point to note is the increase in hair of the eyebrows and head.

may therefore present in a manner indistinguishable from primary hypo-thyroidism. Clinical features suggesting an adenohypophysial origin (when signs of adrenocorticotrophin deficiency are absent) are a thin pale skin, and the absence of pubic and axillary hair. Symptoms and signs of the underlying adenohypophysial lesion may also be present (see Chapter 2). It is important to remember that minor degrees of adrenocortical deficiency may become apparent when thyroid replacement therapy is given, and an adrenal crisis can be precipitated.

INVESTIGATION: Thyroid hormone measurements are often sufficient for diagnosis. TSH levels will then help to differentiate primary from secondary disease and assist in the assessment of equivocal thyroid hormone results. The significance of slightly raised plasma TSH with normal circulating thyroxine levels (premyxoedema,† compensated hypothyroidism, subclinical hypo-thyroidism) is still under review.

Several associated abnormalities may be found on investigation. Hyper-cholesterolaemia is not necessarily diagnostic of myxoedema, but if the level falls to normal with adequate thyroid therapy then this test assists in estab-lishing that the patient was hypothyroid. Similarly the duration of the relax-ation phase of the Achilles' tendon reflex decreases to normal values. The finding of significant quantities of thyroid antibodies adds some support to the diagnosis of thyroid disease. In addition the following changes may be seen: anaemia (normochromic, normocytic, but occasionally macrocytic), hypo-natraemia, raised serum enzymes, of which creatine kinase (CK) is the most important, increased gamma-globulins, bradycardia, low-voltage complex sometimes with inversion of the T wave of the cardiogram, and cardiomegaly on chest X-ray. The quantity of steroids of adrenal cortical origin secreted in the urine in 24 h is reduced in primary as well as in secondary myxoedema, thus this test fails to differentiate between these two conditions. It is interesting, despite this change, that the plasma cortisol levels may be normal in primary myxoedema, possibly due to the reduced steroid metabolism.

TREATMENT: Thyroid hormone replacement with L-thyroxine is the treatment of choice for primary hypothyroidism. Therapy should start at a low dose of 100 μg daily or even 50 μg in elderly patients with long-standing myxoedema. Dosage can be increased every four weeks either by 100 μg or 50 μg. Once established, treatment must be continued indefinitely and can be monitored by TSH measurements or by the plasma cholesterol level. The mean final dose is 150 μg/day, although at some centres 300 μg are administered. It is claimed that cardiac failure or anginal pain may be precipitated by replacement therapy.

Replacement of thyroid hormone should be given together with glucocor-ticosteroid for several weeks in patients with adenohypophysial disease. Because of the difficulty in separating severe primary hypothyroidism from

---

† Premyxoedema, a condition in which there is a low normal serum thyroxine, a raised or normal basal TSH, but an exaggerated TSH response to TRH and often a raised serum cholesterol; is thought by some writers to be associated with an increased incidence of coronary heart disease. Treatment with thyroxine is thought to decrease the mortality and morbidity from coronary heart disease.

'pituitary' hypothyroidism and because of the tissue effects of long-standing thyroid deprivation some authorities advise steroid cover in all cases of this nature; where the results of TSH assay are rapidly available such cover is less vital. Other long-term pituitary medication must be given as necessary.

Treatment of myxoedema coma is discussed in the section on endocrine emergencies (Chapter 11).

Other disorders

Pretibial myxoedema

This is a localized infiltration of myxoedematous tissue over the front of the shin which may sometimes extend down to the dorsum of the foot. The affected skin is rough and coloured a purple–red, giving it an orange-peel appearance. It is usually associated with the ocular signs of thyrotoxicosis and occasionally with thyroid acropachy which is a subperiostial thickening in the region of the nail-bed, clinically indistinguishable from clubbing of the fingers. This condition occurs most commonly in hyperthyroidism but is occasionally associated with a hypo- or euthyroid state.

Ophthalmic Graves' disease

The association of thyrotoxicosis with enlargement of the thyroid and typical eye changes can be referred to as Graves' disease. When the eye changes are present in the absence of thyrotoxicosis, in the absence of thyrotoxicosis, it is called ophthalmic Graves' disease, provided that there is no past history of hyperthyroidism. The name is applied whether a goitre is present or not. The eye changes including the ophthalmoplegia may be asymmetrical. Exophthalmos, which may be marked, is diagnosed clinically by observing that the sclera is even visible between the lower lid and limbus of the cornea. However the diagnosis can be established only by measuring the forward protrusion of the eyes with an exophthalmometer. This forward protrusion of the eyeballs is due to an increase of fat in the bony orbit and to swelling of the orbital muscles (the muscle showing lymphoid, water, and mucopolysaccharide infiltration). Usually the proptosis does not progress, but occasionally it may threaten vision (malignant exophthalmos). Although the commonest cause of bilateral or even unilateral exophthalmos is Graves' disease or ophthalmic Graves' disease, it must always be distinguished from any tumour of the orbit.

TREATMENT: The condition often requires no specific therapy: minor degrees of irritation may be treated with methyl cellulose eye-drops and lid retraction may be helped by guanethidine eye-drops. Malignant exophthalmos necessitates more drastic therapy involving large doses of steroids or orbital decompression.

Goitre

Goitre is the name applied to an enlarged thyroid gland. Such enlargement may be associated with normal thyroid function ('simple goitre' and carcinoma), hyperfunction (Graves' disease), or with hypofunction (e.g. lymphocytic thyroiditis). Simple goitre occurs in iodine-deficient areas (few in the United Kingdom) and as a result of certain medications such as para-amino salicylic acid and phenylbutazone. Such goitres rarely produce sufficient displacement of other structures (pressure changes) to warrant the removal of the gland; the patient's complaint is usually on cosmetic grounds.

The assessment and management of a goitre are important. A careful history (making a specific enquiry to determine whether pain is present) and examination of the gland is essential. When examining the gland its consistency, symmetry, and size are determined; subsequently tests of thyroid function are employed.

Simple goitres and those more commonly occurring in association with hypo- and hyperfunctioning glands, although often uncomfortable, are not usually painful. When pain is present the common causes are malignant disease, subacute thyroiditis, or haemorrhage into a pre-existing cyst or nodule.

INVESTIGATIONS: Thyroid scanning determines the functional area of the gland, and whether there are ectopic areas of activity. A malignant nodule is usually single and non active ('cold nodule'). A routine T_4 and T_0 plasma level will indicate the activity of the gland.

Thyroiditis

It is unfortunate that a number of unrelated diseases are grouped together under this title. The commonest and most important of these is autoimmune thyroiditis (including lymphocytic and Hashimoto's thyroiditis) in which there is a varying degree of lymphocytic infiltration. The second most common is subacute thyroiditis (de Quervain's thyroiditis). Both disorders occur predominantly in females. Of very rare occurrence are two varieties of acute thyroiditis, viral and bacterial. Another thyroiditis, Riedel's thyroiditis, is uncommon; in this condition there is fibrous infiltration of the thyroid extending beyond the limits of the gland; it may be extremely difficult to differentiate between this condition and carcinoma of the thyroid. Only the subdivision of Hashimoto's thyroiditis and subacute thyroiditis are considered subsequently.

Hashimoto's thyroiditis is a disorder involving the immune system with the presence of very high thyroid antibody titres. Typically it occurs in middle-aged females, with a diffuse painless goitre and usually signs of hypothyroidism, although it may be preceded by a period of hyperthyroidism or euthyroidism.

Subacute thyroiditis presents as an extremely painful thyroid, with the pain often limited to one side of the gland, with an onset either acute (over a few days) or more commonly over 2–3 months. It is thought to be viral in aetiology and self-limiting though full regression often takes several months. Investigations show characteristically high circulating T_4 and T_3 with low radioiodine uptake. Specific thyroid treatment is not required, although occasionally steroid therapy may be given if the disease is prolonged and incapacitating.

Carcinoma

An apparently single nodule in the thyroid raises the possibility of carcinoma particularly when radioactive scanning reveals a 'cold' nodule. Whereas benign nodular enlargement of the thyroid is common, carcinoma is not.

Whether a nodular thyroid predisposes the gland to malignant changes remains unsettled. Whilst thyroidal carcinomata can be divided histologically into several subgroups, they are of little clinical consequence apart from follicular carcinoma, and papillary carcinoma (which is slow growing with relatively good long-term prognosis) and medullary carcinoma. To confirm the diagnosis, an open thyroid biopsy is required. Treatment in all except papillary carcinoma in the elderly (which needs no specific therapy) is total thyroidectomy followed by radio-iodine investigation with subsequent treatment as required. Surgery for anaplastic tumours should be only palliative.

Medullary carcinoma accounts for less than 10 per cent of all thyroid carcinomata. Its cellular origin is from calcitonin secreting C-cells and thereby differs from other thyroid cancers. Calcitonin is secreted in large quantities into the circulation and, if facilities are available for measuring this hormone, high plasma levels are an aid in confirming the diagnosis. Most patients are asymptomatic but some present with extensive watery diarrhoea. The main interest of medullary carcinoma lies in its relationship to other endocrine neoplasms (multiple endocrine adenomatosis Type 2, see Chapter 9).

Familial thyroid disease

In clinical practice, families are occasionally found in which there is a high incidence of thyroid disease. In some cases this is due to common environmental factors (iodine deficiency, ingestion of goitrogens) or to a common predisposition to autoimmune disease (with a high frequency of tissue specific antibodies in unaffected relatives). Alternatively, the finding of thyroid disease in mother and child may result from treatment of the mother during her pregnancy with thyroid hormone or antithyroid medication.

A minority of families exhibit inheritance of a true genetic defect of thyroid hormone synthesis. Several separate defects have been described and are grouped together under the term dys-hormonogeneric goitre. Pendred's syndrome is often used to describe the occurrence of a usually mild iodination defect with goitre and congenital deafness. Patients with dys-hormonogenesis are not usually noticeably affected at birth, but they develop a goitre after a few months to years and, depending upon the severity of the defect, become hypothyroid. Plasma TSH is markedly raised but the identification of the defect involved is a difficult biochemical task.

7 Parathyroids, calcitonin, and calcium metabolism

PHYSIOLOGY

This chapter is concerned with calcium metabolism and the two hormones involved in its regulation, parathormone from the parathyroid glands and calcitonin from the thyroidal parafollicular cells. In addition, vitamin D and its metabolites will be considered briefly since they also play an important role in regulating plasma calcium ion levels.

Anatomy, histology, and development

The parathyroid glands are derived from the third and fourth branchial pouches. In man there are usually four glands, one at each of the superior and inferior poles of the two lobes of the thyroid situated close to the posterior surface. However, the number and the location of the parathyroid glands may vary considerably. Each gland is surrounded by a fibrous capsule through which the blood-vessels and non-medullated nerve fibres penetrate in a distinct stalk; inside the gland arterial blood enters a capillary plexus. There are two types of cell in the gland; the chief cells which synthesize the hormone parathormone, and oxyphilic cells whose function is unknown although they also appear capable of secreting the hormone. The chief cells, which appear at puberty, contain numerous small vesicles associated with the Golgi complex, believed to contain the synthesized hormone, and are considered to represent an initial stage in the formation of larger secretory droplets seen in the cytoplasm. Hyperactivity of the gland is associated with increased numbers of these droplets.

1. Parathormone   Raises plasma Ca⁺⁺

Synthesis, storage, and release

Parathormone (PTH) is a large polypeptide (mol. wt approximately 9500) consisting of 84 amino acids. It is believed to be synthesized initially as part of a precursor molecule called pro-parathormone (mol. wt approximately 12 000) which is present only in small concentrations in the gland. It has less biological and immunological activity than has PTH which is the major secretion of the parathyroid glands; cleavage of the precursor molecule is believed to occur prior to the release.

Actions

Parathormone is probably the most important factor involved in the control of calcium metabolism, and it acts primarily to raise the plasma calcium ion concentration. It also lowers plasma phosphate levels. Its actions are directed at the three organs chiefly involved in calcium metabolism: bone, kidneys, and intestinal tract.

Because calcium ions play a vital role in the regulation of many functions in the body (e.g. altered threshold of nerve excitability) the plasma calcium level is normally maintained within a very small range at approximately 2·5 mmol/l (10 mg/100 ml). Approximately 50 per cent of the plasma calcium is bound to non-diffusible protein, while of the remainder some 1·15 mmol/l are present as freely exchangeable calcium ions and 0·1 mmol/l as diffusible salts such as calcium citrate.

(a) Bone. If the plasma calcium ion level falls, PTH is normally released from the parathyroid glands, its primary target being the principal calcium stores in the body, the bones. Most of the calcium in the bones is in the form of large crystals of hydroxyapatite (a hydrated salt of calcium and phosphate) deposited in the organic matrix. These calcium salts represent about 99 per cent of the total bone calcium and are not readily exchangeable. However the remaining calcium in bone is in the form of an exchangeable salt (probably calcium hydrogen phosphate ($CaHPO_4$)) which forms the major source of readily available calcium. The remaining readily exchangeable calcium comes from other cells of the body, in particular the liver and gastrointestinal tract. The exchangeable calcium component is of great importance because it is in equilibrium with the free calcium ions in the extracellular fluid, and provides a rapid buffering system independent of PTH for sudden changes in plasma calcium levels. It is generally believed that the actions of PTH on bone are involved more in the essential long-term restoration of equilibrium between the extracellular and bone calcium levels than in the immediate response to decrease plasma calcium concentrations.

The hormone has three known effects on bone: (i) stimulation of osteoclastic activity; (ii) the formation of new osteoclasts; (iii) a transient depression of osteoblastic activity. These three effects result in an increased absorption of the bone matrix with the consequent release of calcium which ultimately replaces the readily exchangeable calcium which has been depleted as a result of the more immediate 'buffer action'.

Parathormone exerts these effects by acting on bone cells to increase their intracellular calcium concentration. This alteration of ionic concentration is believed to be due to two separate modes of action of the hormone. The first is a direct membrane mechanism to allow a greater influx of calcium into the cell. This action may account for the puzzling observation that there is a transient decrease in the extracellular calcium concentration a few minutes after the intravenous infusion of PTH. The second is to increase the concentration of intracellular cyclic AMP which may stimulate the movement of calcium ions from the mitochondrial storage sites into the cytoplasm (Fig. 7.1). The resultant increase of cytoplasmic calcium ion concentration is apparently related to the various effects of PTH in the bone cells. These effects may be mediated by the stimulation of DNA synthesis and the production of lysosomal enzymes and other enzymes which may be involved in new cell formation.

In the absence of vitamin D or its metabolites the effect of PTH is greatly reduced; consequently the increase in the cytoplasmic pool of calcium ions is diminished. The increased intracellular calcium ion level would therefore

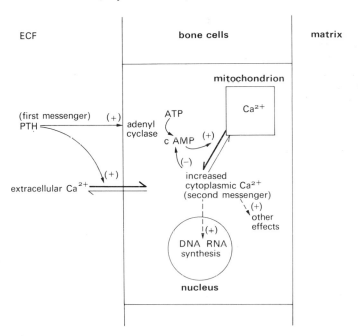

Fig.7.1 Possible mechanisms of action of parathormone (PTH) which result in an increased cytoplasmic calcium ion concentration. The effects of the increased cytoplasmic Ca^{2+} concentration are at present unknown but could include a stimulation of protein synthesis in the nucleus and/or other effects such as the rupturing of lysosomal membranes.

appear to act as a 'second messenger' (PTH being the first messenger) which acts by initiating certain reactions, possibly involving protein synthesis.

(b) Kidneys. The first observed renal action of parathormone is increased phosphate excretion. Originally this renal effect on phosphate was believed to account entirely for the increase in plasma calcium levels since an increased excretion of phosphate alters the state of equilibrium between plasma phosphate and calcium ions with calcium phosphate salts such that a greater dissociation of the salts results. However, it is now known that PTH has a direct effect on calcium reabsorption in the kidney, increasing the quantity absorbed. Parathormone also increases the urinary excretion of sodium, potassium, and bicarbonate ions while decreasing the excretion of magnesium ions. In addition ammonium and hydrogen ion excretion is reduced.

In the proximal tubule, PTH inhibits Na^+, Ca^{2+}, and HPO_4^{2-} reabsorption. In the distal tubule, however, the hormone stimulates calcium reabsorption so that net urinary calcium loss is reduced. The increased tubular load of sodium may account for the increased excretion of potassium ions due to stimulation of the sodium–potassium ion exchange mechanism located in the distal convoluted tubules.

In the kidney PTH also stimulates the renal conversion of a vitamin D metabolite called 25-hydroxycholecalciferol (25(OH)D) to 1,25-

dihydroxycholecalciferol $(1,25(OH)_2D)$. Vitamin D and in particular its metabolites are involved in the regulation of plasma calcium ion levels and will be discussed in subsequent sections.

(c) Intestine. Parathormone stimulates the intestinal absorption of calcium but, since this effect takes several hours to develop and is not observed in vitamin D deficient animals, it is generally believed to be mediated by vitamin D metabolites (chiefly $1,25(OH)_2D$). Nevertheless, a direct and specific effect on calcium absorption from the intestine has been reported with high doses of parathormone.

Mechanisms of action

The precise mechanisms of action of parathormone have not yet been completely elucidated; however the stimulation of adenyl cyclase with the subsequent increase in cyclic AMP formation in bone and kidney cells is believed to be one important mechanism involved in raising intracellular calcium ion concentration. The increased cytoplasmic calcium level may then act to induce RNA synthesis which results in the formation of various proteins such as proteolytic enzymes or carrier proteins. The PTH-stimulated conversion of $25(OH)D$ to $1,25(OH)_2D$ in the kidney may also involve the activation of the adenyl cyclase–cyclic AMP system, with the consequent stimulation of those enzymes necessary for hydroxylation.

Control of release

There is an inverse correlation between the plasma calcium concentration in the range of 1–2·5 mmol/l (4–10 mg/100 ml) and parathormone concentrations, indicating that one important factor involved in the stimulation of PTH secretion is hypocalcaemia. Magnesium ions also appear to be necessary for the operation of this negative feedback since parathormone concentrations do not increase when the hypocalcaemia is linked with a severe hypomagnesaemia. Thyrocalcitonin (TCT) also appears to stimulate the release of PTH from the parathyroids, but this effect is noted only when the TCT level is much higher than the normal physiological range, and therefore this effect may not be part of the normal regulatory mechanism. Vitamin D and its metabolites inhibit the release of PTH probably due to direct stimulation of calcium uptake by the cells of the parathyroids; this is interpreted by the parathyroid sensory mechanisms as an increase in plasma calcium level even though this has not in fact changed. Thus this effect indicates that the level of response by the parathyroid cells to changes in plasma calcium concentrations can itself be regulated by vitamin D and its metabolites.

2. Thyrocalcitonin

Thyrocalcitonin TCT is a small polypeptide of 32 amino acids synthesized in the parafollicular cells (C cells) of the thyroid gland. The embryological derivation of the C cells is discussed in Chapter 6.

Actions

The principal known effect of thyrocalcitonin is to decrease plasma calcium levels by actions on bone, kidney, and possibly on the intestine.

(a) Bone. The effects of TCT on bone consist of (i) decreased activity of osteoclasts and osteocytes on bone reabsorption; (ii) increased rate of formation of osteoblasts from osteoclasts; (iii) decreased formation of osteoclasts. These three effects result in a biphasic action for TCT. First, there is a decreased bone resorption, coupled with an increase in bone production as osteoblastic formation is stimulated, resulting in a positive skeletal balance. This stage may last as long as two months in man. The second stage is due to the gradual decline in the number of osteoclasts which leads in turn to a gradual decrease in the number of osteoblasts; this results in the restoration of skeletal balance to its original level.

Thyrocalcitonin does not block the two cellular effects of PTH, namely the increased uptake of calcium ions from the extracellular fluid and the stimulation of adenyl cyclase. It would therefore appear that the TCT does not act simply by blocking the actions of PTH at the cellular level.

(b) Kidney. In man, thyrocalcitonin infusion results in an increased excretion of sodium, chloride, and calcium, resulting in a saline diuresis which induces a decrease in extracellular fluid volume. It also appears to increase phosphate excretion and inhibits the renal conversion of $25(OH)D$ to $1,25 (OH)_2D$.

(c) Intestine. At present, evidence is generally against an important role for TCT in the regulation of calcium absorption from the gut. However, inhibition of the renal conversion of $25(OH)D$ to $1,25(OH)_2D$ may be of importance in influencing calcium absorption.

Mechanism of action
Observations concerning the mechanism of action of thyrocalcitonin indicate an initial release of calcium ions from bone cells followed by an inhibition of this release. In addition calcitonin may stimulate some unidentified 'second messenger' which then induces mitochondrial calcium retention. The cytoplasmic concentration of calcium falls, this resulting in a removal of the inhibition of adenyl cyclase which the cytoplasmic calcium level is presumed to exert. Indeed, the actions of PTH and TCT both appear to involve increases in the intracellular concentration of cyclic AMP, indicating that while the two hormones may bind initially to different receptors, they do not act antagonistically at the cellular level. The mechanisms of action involved in the stimulation of osteoblastic formation from osteoclasts, and the inhibition of new osteoclastic formation from osteoprogenitor cells by TCT are not yet resolved but they may be on the same pathways as those acted on by PTH (see Fig. 7.2). The mechanism of action of TCT on the kidney has not yet been resolved, but it does not appear to involve cyclic AMP stimulation.

Control of release
The only established physiological control mechanism involved in the regulation of TCT secretion is the plasma calcium level. If this plasma level rises above 2·4 mmol/l (9·5 mg/100 ml) the rate of secretion of TCT rises proportionally. Below this level TCT cannot normally be detected in the adult.

Magnesium ions have also been shown to stimulate TCT secretion from the parafollicular cells, but the concentrations necessary are high and outside the normal physiological range. Another possible regulator of TCT secretion is an

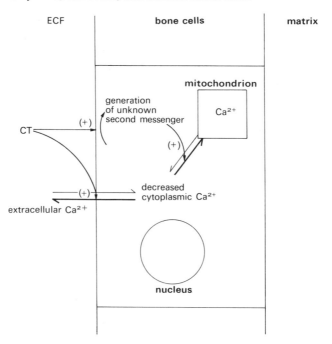

Fig.7.2   Possible mechanisms of action of calcitonin (CT) which result in a decreased cytoplasmic calcium ion concentration. The cellular effects of this decrease are at present obscure.

unidentified hormone from the gastrointestinal tract. In young animals it has been shown that TCT levels in the plasma increase significantly following the intake of a high calcium-content meal without a rise in plasma calcium. While it is possible that the plasma calcium level rises by a very small and undetectable amount, thereby stimulating TCT secretion, it appears more likely that gastrin and pancreozymin may be involved.

3. Vitamin D and its metabolites

The physiological effects of vitamin D (cholecalciferol) on calcium balance are mainly due to the formation of its more potent metabolites. The first of these metabolites is a monohydroxylated form of vitamin D called 25-hydroxycholecalciferol (25(OH)D) which is synthesized mainly in the liver but also in other tissues such as kidneys and intestine. The rate of formation of 25(OH)D is self-limiting so that as the concentration of this metabolite increases it exerts a negative feedback on the hydroxylation process resulting in an increased storage of vitamin D in the liver. Normally the monohydroxy-metabolite is then converted to other hydroxylated forms of vitamin D, the most important biologically being the dihydroxy-metabolite 1,25(OH)$_2$D which is synthesized in the kidneys. The other two metabolites formed are

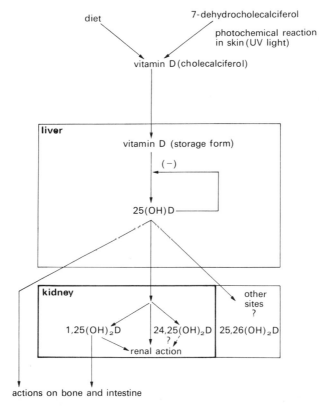

Fig.7.3 The biosynthesis pathway of the various hydroxy-metabolites of vitamin D (cholecalciferol). The renal conversion of 25(OH)D to the dihydroxy-metabolites 1,25(OH)₂D and 24,25(OH)₂D is stimulated by parathormone (PTH) and inhibited by calcitonin (CT).

$24,25(OH)_2D$ and $25,26(OH)_2D$; the first of these is also synthesized in the kidneys but the site of synthesis of the second has not yet been established. These two metabolites do not appear to have much biological activity (see Fig. 7.3).

Actions

Vitamin D, and in particular its two metabolites $25(OH)D$ and $1,25(OH)_2D$, participate in the regulation of plasma calcium ion concentrations by acting on bone, kidneys and intestinal tract.

(a) Bone. Vitamin D metabolites (mainly $1,25(OH)_2D$), maintain the stores of calcium in the mitochondria. When vitamin D is absent the calcium ion stores in the mitochondria are reduced so that the PTH-induced stimulation of cyclic AMP on calcium efflux from the mitochondria is no longer effective. This could account for the observation that in vitamin-D deficiency (e.g.

PTH +Vit D: ↑Ca⁺⁺ ‖Calciton in lower Ca⁺⁺ or

rickets) the effect of PTH in stimulating calcium resorption from bone is greatly reduced, presumably because the cytoplasmic calcium ion concentration is now reduced and so cannot act as 'second messenger'. In hypoparathyroid patients administration of large quantities of vitamin D can cause bone resorption to be increased almost as much as by PTH alone, possibly because the mitochondrial stores of calcium are so enriched that the cytoplasmic calcium levels are consequently increased. The mechanism of action of this effect on the mitochondrial membrane is not yet known but cyclic AMP stimulation does not appear to be involved.

(b) Kidney. Recent studies have indicated that 25(OH)D and 1,25(OH)$_2$D both increase calcium reabsorption from the proximal tubules. The monohydroxy-metabolite appears to be more potent but its action is counteracted by parathormone. The mechanism of action has not yet been elucidated but appears to involve cyclic AMP.

(c) Intestine. The absorption of calcium from the intestine is now believed to be controlled by 25(OH)D and in particular 1,25(OH)$_2$D, so that any effect by PTH is probably indirect, through its action in stimulating the renal conversion of the mono to the dihydroxy-metabolite. Intestinal calcium transport is energy dependent since movement of calcium from lumen to serosa is against a strong electrochemical gradient. The action of 1,25(OH)$_2$D may involve the synthesis of a carrier-protein molecule which can transport calcium ions across the mucosal cell membrane or across the intestinal cell itself. However a membrane-bound calcium-dependent ATPase which is positively correlated with increased calcium transport has also been observed.

Summary

1. The plasma calcium ion concentration is in equilibrium with the bound ion and the principal factor involved in its regulation is PTH from the parathyroid glands. The release of PTH is stimulated by a decrease in the calcium ion level. It acts by increasing bone resorption, increasing calcium reabsorption from the kidneys, and by stimulating the renal conversion of 25-hydroxy-vitamin D to the 1,25-dihydroxy-metabolite.

2. The vitamin D metabolites are necessary for the actions on PTH on bone reabsorption, but also have effects of their own on intestinal calcium absorption and on renal calcium reabsorption.

3. Calcitonin from the parafollicular cells of the thyroid decreases the plasma calcium concentration, but its physiological role in the adult human is debatable.

4. The principal mechanism of control for PTH and calcitonin release appears to be by direct negative feedback from the plasma calcium ion level itself.

By means of these three hormonal systems (assuming vitamin D metabolites to be hormones) the plasma calcium concentrations are finely regulated in the normal state.

CLINICAL DISORDERS

The majority of patients with diseases of the parathyroid glands are investigated in the context of abnormal calcium metabolism. Tables 7.1 and 7.2 outline the differential diagnoses which must be considered when investigating hyper- or hypo-calcaemia respectively. Ionized plasma calcium rather than total plasma calcium is of primary importance. Unfortunately it is difficult to

Table 7.1   Causes of hypercalcaemia

1. Endocrine:
  a. primary, secondary and tertiary hyperparathyroidism
  b. hyperthyroidism (unusual)
  c. adrenocortical insufficiency (rare)

2. Metabolic disturbances:
  d. vitamin D excess
  e. milk–alkali syndrome
  f. sarcoidosis

3. Bone disease:
  g. metastatic carcinoma, myeloma, reticuloses
  h. non-metastatic carcinoma
  i. Paget's disease—immobilized

4. Drugs:
  j. iatrogenic–vitamin B_4; thiazides; ion-exchange resins

Table 7.2   Causes of hypocalcaemia

1. With normal ionized calcium:
  a. hypoproteinaemia:
    i.   nephrotic syndrome
    ii. hepatic cirrhosis
    iii. (severe) malnutrition
  b. renal failure

2. With reduced ionized calcium:
  a. Endocrine—hypoparathyroidism:
    i.   true:
        Iatrogenic
        Autoimmune
        Idiopathic
    ii. false:
        pseudohypoparathyroidism
  b. vitamin D abnormalities—dietary:
    i.   malabsorption—gastrointestinal disease
    ii. anticonvulsants
    iii. renal failure
  c. other causes such as acute pancreatitis

measure ionized calcium and this test is therefore rarely available in clinical practice. A variety of formulae dependent upon plasma proteins and pH have been described to derive a value for unbound calcium (and hence ionized calcium) from the total level. For accurate assessment, blood samples for calcium determinations must be collected under strict conditions. Ideally the patient should be fasting and have been at rest for 30 min. The sample is then collected without the stasis caused by a tourniquet.

Parathormone

Excess

Increased secretion of parathormone may be due to a disorder of the parathyroid glands (primary hyperparathyroidism) or be a compensating mechanism secondary to low plasma calcium (secondary hyperparathyroidism).

Most patients with hypercalcaemia do not have hyperparathyroidism, but may have one of the alternative diseases listed in Table 7.1. Amongst those found to have parathyroid disease the vast majority (over 85 per cent) will have a single 'autonomous' adenoma. Only a small number will have multiple adenoma (about 3 per cent), hyperplasia of all parathyroids (about 7 per cent) or carcinoma (about 3·5 per cent).

Primary hyperparathyroidism

All patients with renal stones should be investigated for hyperparathyroidism although only a minority will have excess parathyroid hormone secretion, as hyperparathyroidism is a rare disease.

CLINICAL FEATURES: By far the commonest presentation is some renal disorder—stone formation, nephrocalcinosis or less commonly tubular dysfunction with polyuria, inability to concentrate urine, hypokalaemia, and acidosis. Gastrointestinal symptoms may be due to the high incidence of peptic ulcer in this disease, to non-specific dyspepsia, or to associated pancreatitis. High plasma calcium levels can induce gastrin secretion but whether this is of sufficient magnitude to produce symptoms remains uncertain. 'Hypercalcaemic crisis' with a high plasma calcium level and impairment of consciousness is rarely due to hyperparathyroidism, but since a high concentration of this ion may be lethal the early recognition and treatment of this condition is essential (Chapter 11). Mental changes may occur and occasionally the patient may be believed to be suffering from a psychotic episode. Table 7.3 briefly summarizes the incidence of the clinical manifestations.

Clinical examination contributes very little towards the diagnosis of hyperparathyroidism. Although a lump may be found in the neck, it is usually of thyroid origin and not parathyroid. Corneal calcification is a relatively common sign (25 per cent), but careful examination is required for its detection.

INVESTIGATIONS: The presence of hypercalcaemia and significant hypercalciuria are the tests initially performed in the diagnosis of hyperparathyroidism. In view of the problems of sampling and of interpreting total plasma calcium estimations, at least three specimens are obtained under standard conditions. Hyperchloraemic acidosis in the presence of a raised plasma calcium concentration supports the diagnosis of hyperparathyroidism.

Table 7.3 **Presentation of hyperparathyroidism**

	Percentage of cases
Renal stones and nephrocal cinosis	47
Bone disease	13
Gastrointestinal manifestations	12
Symptoms of hypercalcaemia (anorexia, fatigue, polyuria)	7
Hypertension	4
Psychiatric disorders	2
Accidental	8
Others	7

Reproduced from Watson (1974). Hyperparathyroidism. In *Clinics in Endocrinology and Metabolism*, by kind permission of the author and publishers, W. B. Saunders & Co. Limited.

The finding of hypercalcaemia in the absence of hypercalciuria is evidence in favour of some other cause for the hypercalcaemia, namely the milk–alkali syndrome, renal tubular acidosis, etc.

It is now possible to obtain measurements of the plasma parathormone concentration in most biochemical laboratories. If the hormone and plasma calcium levels are raised these provide sufficient evidence for the diagnosis of hyperparathyroidism in most cases. Investigations for other causes of hypercalcaemia or for ectopic production of parathyroid hormone must be carried out in an appropriate manner in each patient.

If the blood alkaline phosphatase is raised, radiological examination may be of value to establish the presence of osteitis fibrosa. X-rays of the hand show the typical subperiosteal erosions of the middle and terminal phalanges. The traditional skull X-rays revealing cystic lesions and loss of the lamina dura are classical changes observed in hyperparathyroidism.

TREATMENT: The natural history of asymptomatic primary hyperparathyroidism is at present still under review. Until this is complete the dilemma over management of the increasing number of patients found in this category will remain.

When symptoms are present the treatment is surgical removal of the abnormal tissue provided the patient is fit for operation. Hypercalcaemic crisis should be controlled before operation is contemplated (see Chapter 11). Local excision of adenomata, subtotal resection for generalized hyperplasia, or extensive resection followed by radiotherapy for carcinoma, are required. Operation is made more difficult by the considerable variation in both number and position of the parathyroid glands all of which should be identified during the procedure. In attempts to overcome these difficulties various pre-operative techniques for the localization of normal and abnormal parathyroid tissue have been employed. Parathormone levels in samples collected by selective venous sampling (i.e. collected by catheterizing separately the veins draining the area) appears to have given the best results. Barium swallow with lateral views on screening, arteriography, staining of parathyroid tissue by pre-operative methylene-blue infusion, or radio-isotope scanning are occasionally helpful.

Most patients develop transient hypocalcaemia postoperatively. Careful postoperative supervision is required to record symptoms of neuromuscular depression and parasthesiae; repeated examination for Chvostek's sign (irritability of facial nerve) and Trousseau's sign (carpopedal spasm within 3–5 min of inducing ischaemia) are important. If these signs occur, slow intra-venous administration of calcium gluconate (20 ml of 20% solution) is required, and this may have to be repeated. Further problems can be avoided by increasing calcium intake with additional dihydrotachysterol. These supplements may need to be continued for 2–3 months after which they should be discontinued in order to reassess the clinical state.

After the immediate postoperative period the development of hypoparathyroidism still remains the major complication of parathyroid surgery. Recurrence of hyperparathyroidism (due usually to inadequate initial surgery) requires a second neck exploration which is exceedingly difficult and is not always satisfactory.

Secondary hyperparathyroidism

Secretion of parathormone is increased as a normal homeostatic response when the free plasma calcium concentration is low. Such a situation occurs in renal failure, intestinal malabsorption, vitamin D and calcium deficiencies, pregnancy, and lactation. The biochemical findings and parathyroid hormone plasma assays usually establish the diagnosis. As the parathyroid glands are responding in a normal manner, only the underlying condition must be appropriately treated.

Tertiary hyperparathyroidism

This term is usually applied to the development of an apparently autonomous parathyroid adenoma after long-standing hyperactivity due to secondary hyperparathyroidism. Some authorities have unfortunately used different criteria to define the term.

An adenoma may develop particularly in the hyperplastic glands secondary to renal failure, malabsorption, or chronic vitamin D deficiency. Plasma calcium, normally reduced in these conditions, may therefore still be in the normal range in the presence of autonomous excess secretion of parathyroid hormone. Ectopic calcification may result and further aggravate any renal failure.

Treatment in these cases is the same as for primary hyperparathyroidism; however, the underlying nature of the illness may result in a poor prognosis.

Deficiency

An abnormally low secretion of parathormone (hypoparathyroidism) is usually consequent upon surgical damage to the parathyroids or their complete removal. The remaining cases include congenital absence of parathyroid glands, autoimmune disease, and possibly an idiopathic variety (Table 7.2).

Magnesium deficiency is a rare cause of a functional reversible hypo-parathyroidism.

CLINICAL FEATURES: Patients with hypocalcaemia from whatever cause (see Table 7.2) most commonly present with manifestations of tetany (apparent or latent) or with epilepsy. Epileptic seizures due to hypocalcaemia are indistinguishable from those due to other causes. Latent tetany may be accompanied by symptoms of parasthesiae or muscle cramps. Untreated hypocalcaemia will lead after several years to changes in personality and intelligence.

Careful examination for neuromuscular irritability, i.e. latent tetany (generalized increased reflexes, Chvostek's and Trousseau's signs), is the most important part of the clinical assessment. Abnormal dentition, cataracts, or papilloedema may be found. The cause of the last is unknown and may be misleading in the presence of epileptiform fits, which would usually indicate a varied intracracial pressure.

INVESTIGATIONS: Low levels of plasma calcium and parathormone confirm the diagnosis in the absence of a magnesium deficiency. If, following the administration of PTH, there is an increase of serum calcium (or phos-phaturia) then a magnesium deficiency cannot be responsible for the biochem-ical changes. Additional investigations may show basal ganglia calcification on skull X-ray and an increased QT_c interval on the cardiogram (see Chapter 11).

TREATMENT: Pure human parathormone is not available for treatment and resistance rapidly develops to treatment with bovine hormone. The admin-istration of large doses of vitamin D (about 2 mg daily) is the standard long-term medication, although the more recently issued vitamin D metabo-lites may be more potent. Patients with only partial hypoparathyroidism can be treated with calcium supplements alone. Acute hypocalcaemia (tetany, epilep-tiform fits) must be treated immediately with intravenous calcium gluconate (Chapter 11).

Pseudohypoparathyroidism

This disorder presents with those changes indicated by hypocalcaemia; it occurs in a younger age group (about 8 years of age) than in idiopathic hypoparathyroidism (about 17 years of age). It is a sex-linked, dominantly inherited disorder with typical somatic features of short stocky build, round face, abnormal fourth and fifth metacarpals, and subnormal intelligence. Ectopic calcification, including subcutaneous calcification, is much more common than in idiopathic hypoparathyroidism.

Pseudohypoparathyroidism is not really a disease of the parathyroid glands for circulating levels of parathormone are high and are suppressible by calcium infusions (i.e. analogous to secondary hyperparathyroidism). Instead, it is due to an end-organ resistance to the hormone, and following the administration of parathyroid hormone, the expected increase in urinary excretion of cyclic AMP is absent. However, there is evidence that this condition is made up of a family of disorders; for example, some patients respond to exogenous para-thyroid hormone suggesting that in these cases the endogenous hormone is itself inactive. Patients may be treated with calcium supplements and vitamin D.

Pseudopseudohypoparathyroidism

Patients with this disorder are phenotypically the same as those with pseudohypoparathyroidism (to whom they may be related), but they differ in that none of the biochemical abnormalities are present and parathyroid hormone levels are normal. They are accordingly asymptomatic apart from the occasional occurrence of hypocalcaemia under conditions of calcium stress.

8 The pancreas

PHYSIOLOGY

The pancreas has both an exocrine and an endocrine function. The latter function is limited to the islets of glandular tissue first described by Langerhans in 1869. The islets form less than 2 per cent of the pancreatic tissue, but their endocrine secretions nevertheless play an important role in regulating the blood glucose concentration. The two principal hormones produced from the islet cells are insulin and glucagon, both of which will be discussed in this chapter.

Anatomy, histology, and development

The pancreas develops from the endoderm of the foregut close to the junction with the midgut; a dorsal and a ventral outgrowth form a typical exocrine gland connected by ducts to the gut. Cells bud off from the duct system to form isolated clumps which are the islets of Langerhans. These are embedded in the exocrine tissue of the pancreas which receives its arterial blood-supply from the splenic, hepatic, and superior mesenteric arteries. Venous blood drains into the splenic and superior mesenteric veins. Nerve fibres to the pancreas appear to terminate on islet cells as well as on exocrine tissue cells. In man, three types of cell have been identified in the endocrine pancreas, and these are called α-, β-, and δ- cells. The α- and β-cells synthesize and secrete the hormones glucagon and insulin respectively; the δ-cells have no clearly defined physiological function although it seems possible that they secrete gastrin (see Chapter 9) and/or somatostatin (somatotrophin release-inhibiting factor). All three types of cell contain secretory granules. Both the α- and β-cells have high concentrations of round granules, the α-cells having large dense centres and the β-cells appearing to contain a few 'crystals'. The δ-cells have numerous closely packed granules which are less dense than those of the other two types of cell. The α- and β-cells appear to be linked together by junctions which implies that the cells may act together in a close relationship to control glucose homeostasis. Somatostatin from the δ-cells has also recently been implicated in the regulation of both insulin and glucagon release. Unmyelinated sympathetic and parasympathetic nerve fibres are in close association with all three cell types. The islets are surrounded by basement membranes separate from the capillary membranes, and when hormones are released from any particular group of cells in the islets, they have to cross these two membranes before entering the blood-stream.

The hormones of the pancreas

1. Insulin

Synthesis, storage, and release

It is probable that insulin is synthesized initially in the form of a precursor molecule called proinsulin on ribosomes along the endoplasmic reticulum of the β-cells. Human proinsulin is a single chain polypeptide containing 86 amino acids (mol. wt 9000) which folds spontaneously upon itself so that disulphide bonds can be formed. The proinsulin molecules are then transported to the Golgi complex where they become incorporated into granules. Once in the granules, proteolysis is believed to occur with the formation of insulin (mol. wt 6000) and a cleavage peptide (mol. wt 3000). The insulin molecule consists of an A-chain of 21 amino acids, and a B-chain of 30 amino acids. The two chains are linked together by two disulphide bridges. Potency appears to reside in the whole molecule.

The insulin is then stored in the granules in the form of a complex with zinc. The β-cells normally contain a large store of insulin (approximately 200 U in man, which is about ten times the normal daily requirement), and it appears that the synthesis and storage of this hormone are not directly related to release, so that each process is separately regulated. Variations of blood-glucose concentration within the physiological range alter the frequency of action potentials recorded in the β-cells; a rise or fall in the extracellular glucose concentration increases or decreases the frequency respectively. The current view on the mechanism for release of insulin is that a stimulus such as an increased blood-glucose level enhances the intracellular uptake of calcium which is probably associated with the development of action potentials. This increase in intracellular calcium concentration may then trigger some contractile process, possibly involving a microtubular network, so that granules from the cell interior migrate to the cell surface. Another intracellular mechanism which may be concerned in insulin secretion involves an alteration of cyclic AMP concentration which could modulate the response of the islet cell. The ultimate release of insulin into the blood-stream is brought about by the process of exocytosis, in which the membrane of the granule fuses with the cell membrane. Some insulin may however be released by a variety of secondary mechanisms, including the intracellular rupture of granules, or the release of a soluble pool of insulin from the cytoplasm. Some proinsulin is always secreted with the insulin, and approximately 10 per cent of the total insulin-like activity in plasma as determined by radio-immunoassay can be accounted for by this molecular component.

Actions

The principal actions of insulin involve carbohydrate, protein, and fat metabolism and these effects are considered separately. In addition, the action of insulin on the cellular uptake of potassium ions will be briefly discussed. A summary of the principal effects of insulin is given in Table 8.1.

(a) Carbohydrate metabolism. The principal action of insulin is to lower the blood-glucose concentration. The normal arterial blood-glucose level is usually maintained within a range of $4\cdot2$–$6\cdot3$ mmol/l (80–120 mg/100 ml). Insulin

Table 8.1 Some of the actions of insulin

Membrane effects:
1. glucose transport (and some other monosaccharides) increased
2. amino acid transport (especially arginine) increased
3. fatty acid transport increased
4. cellular uptake of K^+ and Mg^{2+} increased†

Intracellular effects:
1. increased RNA and DNA synthesis
2. increased protein synthesis
3. increased stimulation of glycogen synthatase (glycogenolysis)
4. stimulation of glucokinase
5. inhibition of glucose 6-phosphatase
6. stimulation of lipogenesis
7. decreased lipolysis (inhibition of cyclic AMP synthesis)
8. increased nucleic acid synthesis†
9. increased Mg^{2+} activated Na^+–K^+ATPase activity†

† Little is known of the importance of these actions of insulin.

produces its various effects by binding to a cell-membrane receptor, which presumably changes the membrane's kinetics such that various intracellular mechanisms can be induced. One important effect is to increase the peripheral uptake of glucose in such tissues as skeletal muscle, cardiac muscle, and adipose tissue. It is believed that the cell membranes of these tissues are relatively impermeable to glucose molecules in the absence of insulin.

Insulin increases the cellular uptake of glucose provided that a glucose concentration gradient across the membrane is present. Observations such as that of the competition between glucose and galactose provide evidence that transport across the membrane is mediated by a process called facilitated diffusion. This process follows saturation kinetics indicating the presence of a carrier, probably a protein in the membrane, which is activated by insulin. It must be emphasized that even in the absence of insulin, a small quantity of glucose will be able to enter the peripheral cells by simple diffusion, provided that there is a concentration gradient across the cell membrane. In this situation the quantity of glucose which enters the cells by simple diffusion is relatively small even in the presence of a markedly elevated blood-glucose concentration. Since glucose is usually rapidly metabolized to glucose 6-phosphate within the cells, the intracellular glucose concentration is generally very low, with a concentration gradient always being present. Insulin stimulates the activity of the carrier mechanism so that glucose is transferred rapidly across the cell membrane in both directions, the net flux being determined by the concentration gradient.

This action of insulin is absent in the cells of the brain and the liver. The cells of the brain and the liver are dependent upon simple diffusion of glucose and therefore they rely upon the maintenance of normal physiological blood-glucose concentrations. It appears that the active transport mechanism for glucose (associated with sodium) in renal tubular epithelium, intestinal mucosa and erythrocytes is also independent on insulin. One interesting observation concerning this facilitated diffusion is that anoxia, cyanide, or other more specific metabolic inhibitors appear greatly to increase the uptake of glucose (see Chapter 10).

In addition to this effect on glucose uptake by peripheral cells, insulin also has important effects in stimulating anabolic reactions. Glycogen synthesis is stimulated in the liver and other cells, an effect which is independent of the glucose-transport action; and the enzyme glycogen synthetase is stimulated, resulting in an increased incorporation of glycosyl units (formed from uridine diphosphoglycose) into glycogen. In addition it stimulates the activity of hepatic glucokinase, an enzyme which phosphorylates glucose to glucose 6-phosphate. Insulin also inhibits the activity of glucose 6-phosphatase, an enzyme which is present mainly in hepatic tissue (although some is found in the kidney), and which dephosphorylates glucose 6-phosphate so that the free glucose formed can then diffuse out of the liver into the blood.

(b) Protein metabolism. Insulin stimulates the uptake of amino acids by cells, and in addition catalyses the synthesis pathways for new protein. These two effects are independent of each other, the increased uptake being purely a membrane phenomenon, the protein anabolic effect being an action at the nuclear level. Any effect of insulin at the nuclear level cannot be direct since the hormone is generally believed to be unable to pass through the cell membrane. The nuclear effects must therefore be mediated by some, as yet unidentified, intracellular mechanism possibly involving the formation of a second messenger (see Chapter 10). The intracellular effects of insulin on protein synthesis include a stimulation of RNA and in particular messenger RNA. Insulin also stimulates peptide bonding in the microsomes. Partly because of the various effects of insulin on protein synthesis, this hormone plays an important role in the process of growth.

(c) Fat metabolism. The cellular uptake and oxidation of glucose by adipose tissue are enhanced by insulin. These effects, together with a stimulation of lipogenesis in the liver and in adipose tissue, result in the increased storage of energy substrates, principally in the form of fats. It is believed that this hormone also stimulates the uptake of fatty acids by adipose tissue. In addition cholesterologenesis, which takes place mainly in the liver, is stimulated by insulin.

(d) Potassium metabolism. Insulin increases the cellular uptake of potassium ions, this effect possibly being linked to the hormone-stimulated glucose transport mechanism.

Control of secretion

The control of insulin secretion is a difficult subject because of the complexity of the interaction between various factors. This section therefore requires careful consideration.

Insulin is secreted even in the absence of a specific stimulus. This basal secretion of the hormone has been estimated as 0·5 U/h entering the circulation. It is believed that the level of insulin secretion may partly determine the response of the β-cells to a particular stimulus. There is also evidence to suggest that the sympathetic nervous system plays a role in continuously modulating the basal secretion. Stimulation of the sympathetic α-receptors (i.e. by noradrenalin) inhibits the release of insulin so that direct stimulation of the sympathetic nerves to the pancreas can inhibit the insulin release induced by a rise in blood-glucose. However stimulation of the sympathetic β-receptors (adrenalin) probably increases insulin secretion. In circumstances when circulating catecholamines are present, the net effect nevertheless appears to be the inhibition of insulin secretion, and the current view is that the sympathetic nervous system continually modifies the response of β-cells to stimuli that usually result in inhibition of secretion. Conversely parasympathetic activity (or administration of acetycholine) stimulates insulin release, but the part played by this system in the maintenance of glucose homeostasis is unknown.

Following a stimulus for the release of insulin (such as an increase in blood-glucose concentration) there appears to be a biphasic response: there is an immediate (within seconds) secretion of insulin which then gradually decreases, followed by a second, more gradual increase in insulin release which reaches its peak later. The initial increase appears to depend on the basal rate of secretion, on the glucose concentration, and on other factors. The second phase also appears to depend on the blood-glucose concentration. These observations indicate that there are two pools of insulin, only one of which is readily available.

Various substrates are capable of stimulating the release of insulin from the β-cells, and of these the most important substrate is probably glucose. Glucose appears not only to stimulate its release, but also to play some role in the regulation of the basal rate of secretion. It would appear that the β-cell 'recognizes' the glucose molecule through some receptor, and this recognition stimulates insulin release. Other substrates such as amino acids (especially arginine) induce the secretion of insulin, although little is known about their mechanism of action. Fatty acids appear to stimulate the release of insulin only very slightly in man, and therefore play a very minor role in the normal physiological control of its release. It is of interest to note that synergistic effects on insulin secretion have been observed between different substrates, for instance between glucose and amino acids. Other hormones have been shown to stimulate the release of insulin. Glucagon has quite a potent effect in stimulating the β-cells. Certain gastrointestinal hormones, in particular gastrin, secretin, and pancreozymin, all stimulate insulin secretion, which accounts for the observation that a substrate such as glucose given orally has a far more potent effect on insulin release than if given by intravenous infusion. Hormones such as growth hormone (somatotrophin), glucocorticoids, progesterone, and oestrogens apparently stimulate the release of insulin; however at least part of this response is probably indirect, and may be due to the decreased tissue responsiveness to insulin which these hormones induce. Somatostatin (from the δ-cells) has recently been shown to inhibit the release of insulin. Stress has been shown to be associated with an inhibition of insulin secretion (decreased glucose tolerance) perhaps induced by increased sympathetic activity. It is important to emphasize that the principal factor involved in the control of insulin release is the plasma glucose concentration.

Diabetes mellitus
In the relative or total absence of insulin (diabetes mellitus) blood-glucose

concentrations rise, sometimes reaching levels in excess of 35 mmol/l (about 600 mg/100 ml plasma). The renal proximal tubules normally reabsorb all the glucose filtered by the glomeruli unless the blood-level exceeds 10 mmol/l (180 mg/100 ml plasma). The hyperglycaemia of diabetes exceeds this threshold allowing glucose to be excreted in the urine (glycosuria) inducing an osmotic diuresis (polyuria), although the osmotic change induced by the glucose is small. The excessive water loss results in dehydration and thirst.

A net increase in protein catabolism raises amino acid blood-levels, resulting in an enhanced load of these substances to the liver. Here they are de-aminated, and the carbon residues contribute to the formation of glucose (increased gluconeogenesis) which further exacerbates the hyperglycaemia. The protein depletion contributes to the weakness and loss of weight found in this condition.

Lipolysis is stimulated, with a resulting increase in free fatty acid and glycerol concentrations in the blood (the latter enriching the glucose store through gluconeogenesis); in addition it is of interest that the blood cholesterol level may increase, although the reason for this is obscure. An excess of acetyl CoA accumulates in the liver as it cannot be fully utilized in the tricarboxylic acid cycle. It is then converted in enhanced quantities to acetoacetic acid. This substance is reduced to β-hydroxybutyric acid, or is decarboxylated to form acetone; these three substances are called 'ketone bodies'. Thus the pro-duction of ketone bodies increases and the peripheral utilization is unable to cope with this excess; the blood concentration of ketone bodies rises (ketonaemia). Hence the enhanced fat catabolism is responsible for ketonaemia and also contributes to the loss of body weight in diabetes mellitus.

In diabetic coma the body water content falls to low levels; in addition there is sodium loss due to the associated diarrhoea and vomiting. The plasma volume shrinks, resulting in a serious reduction in cardiac output with the attendant cardiological changes. The ketone bodies accumulate in the blood inducing metabolic acidosis with the consequent development of deep and rapid breathing (Kussmaul breathing) this, if present, being one of the diag-nostic signs of diabetic acidosis. In addition, the breath smells of acetone (rotting apples). The ketonaemia also results in ketonuria once the renal threshold for ketone bodies has been exceeded. The excretion of the strong acids depletes the body of sodium (total body sodium), contributing to the acidosis. It is likely that both the volume depletion and the ketonaemia are, wholly or in part, responsible for the coma.

In diabetes the stimulation of the cellular uptake of potassium is decreased and this ion will leak out of the cells in severe dehydration; this should result in an increased plasma potassium concentration. However the plasma potassium level of untreated diabetics may be normal (approximately 5 mmol/l) because of the concomitantly increased urinary excretion of potassium ions due to the diuresis. It must however be remembered that the total body potassium levels will be reduced even though the plasma level may be normal, or even raised in diabetic coma. This point is of particular relevance to the diabetic in hypergly-caemic coma since the infusion of saline to replenish the blood-volume, together with the administration of insulin, can cause a rapid movement of fluid and potassium back into the cells thus producing a severe hypokalaemia which may be lethal. This effect appears to be enhanced by bicarbonate which is sometimes used in the treatment of the acidosis in diabetic hyperglycaemic coma. For this reason, if bicarbonate has to be administered to the comatose diabetic patient, potassium salts are given concurrently (see Chapter 11).

Hypoglycaemia

Insulin excess such as is found in insulinoma (see clinical section) results in a physiological hypoglycaemia which can be defined as a blood-glucose concentration below 2·2 mmol/l (40 mg/100 ml). Functional hypoglycaemia is the name given to a condition observed in individuals who show these low levels of blood-glucose, but only following a carbohydrate meal. Frequently, individuals with functional hypoglycaemia are emotionally labile and may have a family history of diabetes mellitus. Reactive hypoglycaemia is the term applied to those patients with partial gastrectomy who have hypoglycaemia and its symptoms 2–4 hours after eating. This condition is probably induced by the raised secretion of glucagon and other hormones which indirectly or directly stimulate insuline secretion.

2. Glucagon

Synthesis, storage, and release

Glucagon is a polypeptide of 29 amino acids. It is believed that the synthesis of glucagon occurs in the endoplasmic reticulum (possibly involving a precursor proglucagon molecule) followed by transport to the Golgi complex where the hormone is stored in granules in the α-cells. The hormone may then be released into the blood by the process of exocytosis, although the evidence is inconclusive. The basal concentration of glucagon in the plasma is as yet undetermined, partly because of the existence in the plasma of a very effective degradation system and the rapid removal of the hormone by the liver.

Actions

Glucagon exerts effects on carbohydrate, protein, and fat metabolism. It stimulates glycogenolysis in the liver which results in glucose release into the blood-stream. Glucagon increases hepatic gluconeogenesis and ketogenesis, and stimulates protein catabolism. It also stimulates lipase activity (increased lipolysis) in adipose and hepatic tissues, and as a result plasma levels of non-esterified fatty acids increase. Many of the effects of glucagon appear to be mediated by enhancing cyclic AMP activity (see Chapter 10). The physiological importance of glucagon is demonstrated mainly in fasting conditions, when energy substrate levels in the blood need to be maintained.

Control of release

Hyperglycaemia inhibits, while hypoglycaemia stimulates the release of glucagon. There is evidence to suggest that these effects may partly be mediated directly by insulin (and perhaps by somatostatin from the δ-cells) acting on the cell. The release of glucagon during hypoglycaemia has however been shown to be partially inhibited by adrenergic blocking drugs. The general concept that sympathetic stimulation increases glucagon release while simultaneously inhibiting insulin release is therefore becoming increasingly accepted. The intravenous administration of amino acids (in particular arginine) or protein in the diet appears to stimulate glucagon release. Since certain amino acids also stimulate the release of insulin, the concurrent release of both hormones could in certain instances be favourable to the organism. The insulin could promote the synthesis of new protein, while the glucagon could act to maintain the blood-glucose concentration. Some of the gastrointestinal hormones, in particular pancreozymin, are potent stimulators of glucagon release.

The insulin–glucagon molar-ratio

A delicate balance between the plasma concentrations of insulin and glucagon appears to be necessary for the regulation of metabolism. The molar ratio of the two hormones apparently determines the balance between the storage of energy and its mobilization. It has been suggested that a disturbance of the molar ratio might determine the severity of diabetes; in some patients decreased levels of plasma insulin and increased levels of plasma glucagon have been detected.

CLINICAL DISORDERS

Clinical conditions arising from disorders of insulin secretion are considered in two sections: deficiency (diabetes mellitus) and excess (insulinoma). Glucagonoma is also considered briefly, since such a tumour can also induce diabetes mellitus.

Insulin

Excess

Insulinoma

Insulinoma must be considered as one possible cause of spontaneous hypoglycaemia. This is arbitrarily defined as a blood-glucose concentration below 2·2 mmol/l (40 mg/100 ml). Patients with insulinoma present with a wide variety of signs and symptoms. It may be many years before it is realized that the patient, commonly in the care of the neurologist or psychiatrist, has this rare condition.

CLINICAL FEATURES: There may be odd psychological changes which do not conform to the psychiatrist's classification. For example hypoglycaemia may be responsible for sudden bizarre behaviour in otherwise normal people, such as the housewife who unexpectedly undresses at midday. The patient's behaviour may resemble drunkenness or shows signs of confusion or hallucination.

Alternatively, there may be symptoms and signs associated with local neurological disorders. Initially these changes occur most often at midday or in the afternoon, especially if a meal is missed. Subsequently the changes occur predominantly in the morning as the disease progresses. The severity of the hypoglycaemia may be sufficient to induce coma or convulsions (see p. 181), and the diagnosis should be then apparent. Surprisingly, the hunger and weight gain which might be expected are not frequently observed. Those patients who find that sweet food relieves their symptoms do eventually gain weight. Sweating during the hypoglycaemic state, again somewhat unexpectedly, may not be marked. It is important to be aware of the possibility of this diagnosis in any patient showing episodic changes of pattern in behaviour or neurological disorders, especially if related to the omission of a meal.

INVESTIGATION:

1. an extended oral glucose tolerance test is carried out over 4 hours, as low levels may not occur until this period.

2. a 48-hour fast can be carried out only under supervision with plasma glucose estimations being made every 3 hours. If symptoms occur they must be present at the time when the blood-glucose levels are low and alleviated by glucose administration. By the forty-eighth hour, the blood glucose should reach 2·2 mmol/l (40 mg/100 ml). Very occasionally, it is necessary to extend the fast for another 24 hours to observe this level.

3. following the intravenous administration of 1 mg of glucagon the blood-glucose is estimated every 15 minutes. In the normal patient it should reach a peak at about 30 minutes, returning to approximately the fasting level in about 2 hours. In patients with insulinoma the blood-glucose, after the initial rise, falls below 2·8 mmol/l (50 mg per 100 ml) for periods of up to 3 hours after the injection. An alternative test is to measure plasma insulin, which rises to 150 mU/l, 5 minutes after the injection in patients with insulinoma.

4. immunoassay: the plasma level of insulin must be measured in conjunction with the blood-glucose. The important finding to be made here is an inappropriately high plasma insulin level with respect to the observed plasma-glucose concentration.

5. a coeliac arteriogram may in some cases be justified if there is evidence of an islet cell tumour.

TREATMENT: Treatment is by surgical removal of the tumour. However this is not always easy, as the tumours may be small and/or multiple. Occasionally the tumour may be ectopically situated in the hilum of the spleen or in the wall of the duodenum. If a Meckel's diverticulum is present it may occur in this structure. A careful inspection and, if need be, a dissection is required. If no tumour can be identified, this should be followed by biopsy and examination of frozen sections of the pancreas despite the probable postoperative complications. If under these circumstances a tumour cannot be located, it is probably wiser to avoid any further surgery. The patient is then treated medically with diazoxide (5–15 mg/kg body weight/24 h given orally). With this dose side-effects such as severe hypotension, nausea, or vomiting are avoided. The hyperglycaemia induced by this drug is enhanced, and adverse effects are reduced by the addition of chlorothiazide.

Deficiency

Diabetes mellitus

Although diabetes mellitus should probably be regarded as a generic term comprising a number of syndromes, it is customary to define it as a chronic disorder of carbohydrate, fat, and protein metabolism characterized by hyperglycaemia and commonly glycosuria, caused by a relative or absolute deficiency of insulin. This, considered by some to be the most common endocrine abnormality, has an incidence of about 1–2 per cent in the population. The diagnosis is usually made on the basis of certain symptoms associated with glycosuria and a random blood-glucose concentration in excess of 10·0 mmol/l (180 mg/100 ml), or 6 mmol/l (108 mg/100 ml) in the fasting state. In patients in whom these figures are not exceeded but in whom diabetes mellitus is suspected, it may be necessary to carry out a standard or modified glucose tolerance test (GTT, Chapter 12). Recent work has indicated that diabetes mellitus may have a multifactorial aetiology and this may eventually provide a better understanding of the disease.

Clinical disease is not always evident and the British Diabetic Association has suggested that the following classification be used:

1. Potential (increased tendency to diabetes; no symptoms; normal GTT)

2. Latent (normal GTT, but abnormal under stress; no symptoms)

3. Asymptomatic; sub-clinical or chemical (no symptoms, but abnormal GTT)

4. Clinical.

A convenient subclassification separates clinical diabetes into two distinct categories: (a) juvenile-onset diabetes (JOD), which is insulin dependent; and (b) maturity-onset diabetes (MOD), which is insulin independent. However this classification is not rigid and the two categories overlap. Insulin-dependent diabetes may develop late in life, and recently diabetes in the young has been described which can be controlled without insulin (maturity-onset diabetes of youth, MODY).

It will be seen from Table 8.2 that disorders of carbohydrate metabolism are associated with many endocrine disorders and reference should be made to the relevant chapters when reading this section.

AETIOLOGY: Much interesting work has been done recently in an attempt to identify the fundamental factors which cause diabetes mellitus.

(a) Heredity. It is generally accepted that a genetic factor is in part responsible for the development of diabetes. For example, MODY is believed to be inherited as a Mendelian dominant characteristic. However the importance of heredity in the other types of diabetes is uncertain. While it has been shown that in young insulin-dependent patients (JOD) there is a significant association with certain histocompatible antigens, namely HL–A B8 and Bw18, no such association has been found between insulin-independent diabetics (MOD).

(b) Autoimmunity. As there may be an association between diabetes and pernicious anaemia, Addison's disease, or thyroid disorders, it has been

Table 8.2 Conditions resulting in diabetes mellitus

1. Endocrine:
   a. Relative or absolute deficiency of insulin*
   b. Acromegaly (excess somatotrophin)
   c. Cushing's syndrome (excess cortisol)
   d. Thyrotoxicosis (excess thyroxine)
   e. Phaeochromocytoma (excess adrenalin)
   f. Glucagonoma (excess glucagon)*

2. Drug-induced:
   a. Contraceptive pill
   b. Thiazides
   c. Steroids

3. Other conditions:
   a. Pancreatitis (acute and chronic)
   b. Haemochromatosis

---

* These endocrine conditions are discussed in this chapter. It is probable that the development of diabetes due to the other endocrine disorders or following certain drug therapies occurs only in predisposed subjects.

suggested that all these conditions are autoimmune diseases. Both the presence of islet-cell antibodies in cases of recent onset, and the autopsy finding of 'insulitis' in patients dying soon after the onset of diabetes, suggest a cellular autoimmune response.

(c) Infection. In children, diabetes may follow viral infections such as mumps. It has also been noted that the incidence of diabetes rises with outbreaks of Coxsackie B Infections. It is therefore possible that young people inheriting a particular complex of immune response genes by virtue of their HL–A types could respond to viral infections by initiating an autoimmune process culminating in damage to the islet cells.

CLINICAL FEATURES: Usually the history is a short one with thirst, polyuria, loss of weight, and tiredness being the principal features. Weight is lost despite a good appetite. Pruritus vulvae is common in women and balanitis may occur in men. Infections and skin sepsis often lead to examination of the urine and the discovery of glycosuria. Rarely the presenting symptoms are amenorrhoea, impotence, or blurring of vision resulting either from a change in the refractive index of the lens or, more seriously, from a retinopathy. Glycosuria is increasingly being discovered on routine medical examination for jobs or for insurance. Paradoxically symptoms of hypoglycaemia before meals may on occasion be a prelude to overt diabetes.

At an early stage, there may be little to find apart from the glycosuria. Subsequently the patient may lose weight and show signs of dehydration and a coated tongue. There is infrequently monilial infection of the mouth, pharynx, or vulva, but boils and carbuncles may be troublesome. Maturity onset diabetics are often obese. Sometimes serious complications such as retinopathy, neuropathy, and nephropathy are present at the initial examination and these complications will therefore be considered in some detail. In a few patients the first indication of the disease is coma from hyperglycaemia which is considered in Chapter 11. It is essential that variations in blood-glucose outside the normal range be avoided in all patients with the complications of diabetes.

COMPLICATIONS:

(a) Diabetic retinopathy. This is now the commonest cause of blindness in the United Kingdom in people under the age of 65. The development of retinopathy depends more on the duration of the disease than on its severity, and as a general rule this applies to all the complications of diabetes. The capillaries are affected first, with the formation of microaneurysms recognized as small red dots on ophthalmoscopy. These may rupture, and are then seen as 'blots' when deep, and flame-shaped when superficial. In the macular region 'hard' yellow exudates are often observed, while 'soft' white exudates may be scattered over the retina, these often disappearing within a few weeks. Veins may become nodular and dilated. The formation of new vessels which tend to rupture easily and which extend into the vitreous humour constitutes proliferative retinopathy. Haemorrhage may occur into the vitreous humour and glial formation may follow. The subsequent contraction of fibrous tissue may cause retinal detachment.

Treatment: Coclolfibrate may help to clear exudates speedily, but there is a tendency to recurrence and the long-term effect in preventing the deterioration of vision is limited. Pituitary ablation by surgery or radioactive yttrium was introduced when it was found that retinopathy was halted in cases of pituitary necrosis. At present photocoagulation by laser beam (argon or xenon) is more widely used, as this technique enables the new vessels to be destroyed.

(b) Nephropathy. This is often associated with retinopathy, both being manifestations of an underlying microangiopathy which consists of changes in the basement membrane. Clinically, intermittent or persistent proteinuria becomes evident and oedema may occur. Renal failure indicated by diminished creatinine clearance, high blood-urea levels, and hypertension usually develops. Histologically the glomerular lesions may be diffuse, nodular (Kimmelstiel–Wilson lesion), exudative, or hyaline. These changes may coexist. Fig. 8.1 gives the factors that may eventually result in renal failure.

The kidney is particularly susceptible to infection, either blood-borne or secondary to the 'diabetic bladder' (a result of autonomic neuropathy) with urinary retention and ascending infection. Renal papillary necrosis, also a result of infection, may occasionally occur.

Treatment: There is no specific treatment for this condition. Pituitary ablation may improve the clinical state. Whether dialysis should be used in these patients is debatable, as improvement may not be maintained. Renal transplants have been undertaken with some success.

Pyelonephritis

↓

Arteriosclerosis ⟶ Renal failure ⟵ Glomerular lesions

Fig. 8.1   Factors in diabetes leading to renal failure

(c) Neuropathy. It has been suggested that the fundamental alteration in diabetic neuropathy is segmental demyelination following damage to the Schwann cells. Another factor may be vascular, caused by a microangiopathy of the vasa nervorum. A useful practical classification is as follows:

1. Symmetrical polyneuropathy:
   a. sensory
   b. autonomic
2. Mononeuropathy and multiple mononeuropathy:
   a. cranial nerve lesions
   b. isolated peripheral nerve lesions
   c. 'diabetic amyotrophy'

The symptoms are typical of peripheral nerve damage. Numbness, tingling, and ill-defined pains in the legs at night may be distressing, but there may not be objective signs. The significance of absent vibration sense and ankle jerks is difficult to assess as such changes are found in many healthy elderly people. In more severe cases there is extensive sensory loss such as patchy loss of fine touch in the legs and feet, or sensory loss of the 'glove and stocking' variety; damage to proprioceptive afferent fibres causes ataxia. The motor nerve system may also be involved. Isolated cranial nerve lesions usually affect the third, sixth, or seventh nerves, while an isolated motor mononeuropathy may be manifested as a sudden foot drop. Trophic ulcers in the feet may occur; more rarely neuropathic joints in the feet develop. The autonomic system may be affected throughout the body (Table 8.3). Extensive asymmetrical weakness and wasting of the proximal limb muscles, especially in the legs, may lead to serious disability, for example extreme difficulty in walking. This condition is known as diabetic amyotrophy.

Treatment: Skilful physiotherapy may sometimes produce surprisingly good results by helping patients walk independently. However, there is rarely any improvement of the neuropathic changes.

Table 8.3   Changes produced by malfunction of the autonomic nervous system

Postural hypotension

Abnormalities of sweating

Persistent tachycardia

Derangement of gastrointestinal functions (oesphageal achalasia, atonic dilatation of stomach, epigastric pain, distension, vomiting, and diarrhoea)

Atony of the bladder (straining, dribbling, overflow, incontinence)

Impotence

(d) Diabetic foot. This is a common and troublesome complication, especially in the elderly. There are three elements concerned: (a) neuropathy, (b) arteriopathy, (c) sepsis. As a result of neuropathy there is loss of sensation, particularly over the prominences and callosities of the feet (usually the sole or one of the toes). Patients unwittingly sustain burns or other injuries. Arteriopathy affects the distal vessels such as those of the digits, although the

dorsalis pedis and the posterior tibial arteries may be pulsating strongly. Finally, sepsis supervenes and an infected ulcer develops; this may penetrate to the bone involving the metatarso-phalangeal and interphalangeal joints (neuropathic ulcer).

Arteriosclerosis, which may affect the small blood-vessels in particular, tends to occur at a relatively early age in diabetic patients. These vascular changes may result in ischaemic ulceration of the feet which must be distinguished from neuropathic ulceration, since the latter may respond to conservative treatment. The ischaemic ulceration is at risk of becoming gangrenous.

Treatment: Conservative treatment and patience are all-important – antiseptic dressings are used until the foot is clean, and local surgical toilet may be needed when infection is more widespread. Sometimes one or more toes have to be removed. It may be several months before healing takes place, but encouragingly good results can be obtained. Arterial surgery for diabetic arteriosclerosis is less successful than in non-diabetic patients because of the involvement of small vessels, and amputation may be necessary.

It is essential that diabetic patients pay special attention to their feet. They must be advised about the necessity of comfortable footwear which exerts no abnormal pressure or friction. The feet should be kept clean and dry. Nails and callosities must be treated most carefully, preferably by a qualified chiropodist. Patients must be warned of the danger of unnoticed burns from hot water bottles, electric fires, etc. Minor injuries and sepsis must be treated immediately.

(e) Skin lesions. Boils and carbuncles are said to be more common in diabetics than in healthy individuals but this is debatable. A characteristic skin lesion is necrobiosis diabeticorum, usually occurring on the shins.

Treatment: The treatment of skin infection is standard. It is probably wise to use antibiotics more readily in these patients.

Although not a complication of diabetes mellitus, tuberculosis is more prevalent among diabetics and there may be a relationship between these two conditions. Thus tuberculosis must be considered as a possible cause of any deterioration of the diabetic state, 'general ill health', or chronic cough in a patient with diabetes.

INVESTIGATIONS: The diagnosis of diabetes mellitus is made if the fasting blood-glucose exceeds 6·0 mmol/l (108 mg/100 ml) in the fasting state; in any doubtful case a standard or modified glucose tolerance curve is necessary (Chapter 12). Glycosuria along does not establish the diagnosis of diabetes as it is also found in patients with a low renal threshold for glucose (blood-glucose levels will then be normal). These patients are no more likely to develop diabetes than the rest of the population. In the occasional patient the blood-glucose concentration following the intake of glucose may have a peak greater than normal, although he or she is not diabetic (Chapter 12).

TREATMENT: The three basic considerations in the treatment of diabetes mellitus are described below.

(a) Diet. The overweight maturity-onset diabetic requires a reducing diet of

800–1200 calories (3·4–5 kJ), containing about 100 g of carbohydrate. A diet of 1200–1800 calories (5–7·5 kJ) with 120–180 g carbohydrate is suitable for a patient of average weight. In the young diabetic allowance must be made for growth and activity; the carbohydrate allowance can therefore be increased to 250 g a day. Children who are on insulin therapy are allowed a free diet without carbohydrate restriction by some physicians, but control of the diabetes is more difficult in these cases.

Thus limitation of the carbohydrate intake is generally desirable, although occasionally one must dissuade anxious and obsessive patients from reducing their intake to a harmful level. It has recently been suggested that the carbohydrate content of a diabetic diet could be increased beyond the present customary level in adults provided that the total calorie content was not exceeded. In general the diet should be formulated for each individual to suit his personal taste and cultural habits as well as his clinical need. The advice of an experienced dietitian is invaluable.

(b) Oral hypoglycaemic agents. Diet alone may not be sufficient and oral hypoglycaemic agents may be necessary. However only a minority of juvenile diabetics can be controlled in this way. The oral hypoglycaemic drugs in general use are: (a) the sulphonylureas and (b) the biguanides.

The *sulphonylureas* act by stimulating any residual capacity of the β-cells of the islets to produce insulin. The biguanides delay the absorption of glucose from the gut, increase the uptake of glucose by the muscle cells, and inhibit gluconeogenesis in the liver.

Of the sulphonylureas, tolbutamide, chlorpropamide, and glibenclamide are most commonly used. Tolbutamide acts for a few hours and is given two to three times a day to a total of 0·5–3·0 g; chlorpropamide (100–500 mg) and glibenclamide (2·5–20 mg) are each given as a single daily dose. The sulphonylureas, particularly those with a long-lasting action, can cause hypoglycaemia in the elderly who live alone and who may neglect their diet. There is a tendency to flush after alcohol in patients who are on chlorpropamide, but this is less marked with glibenclamide. The biguanides, phenformin (50–150 mg daily) and metformin (1–1·7 g daily) are given in divided doses two or three times a day; if gastrointestinal disturbance occurs, slow-release capsules are used. At one time phenformin was favoured as it was thought to promote weight reduction in the obese diabetic, but this has proved disappointing. Greater awareness of the danger of lactic acidosis occurring during phenformin therapy has made this drug unpopular and the related biguanide, metformin, is now preferred as possibly a safer though perhaps less effective alternative.

It should be emphasized that oral hypoglycaemic agents have no place in the treatment of ketoacidosis.

(c) Insulin. Severe cases of diabetes require insulin therapy. There is a bewildering variety of insulins and some knowledge of their individual characteristics is necessary. Although each physician may have a preference for certain types, he will inevitably have to deal with patients already on treatment prescribed by others. He must therefore be conversant with them all (see Tables 8.4 and 8.5). Table 8.4 is intended only for the student who may wish to have more detailed information about the insulins.

Table 8.4 Commonly used insulin preparations and their administration

Preparation	Source	Physical state	Retarding principle	pH	Increase of initial effect by addition of:	Frequency of administration
Insulin injection†	Beef‡	Solution		3		Twice or more daily
Actrapid MC	Pig	Solution		7		Twice or more daily
Semilente	Pig	Suspension	Amorphous precipitate of insulin + zinc	7		Twice daily
Semitard MC	Pig	Suspension	Amorphous precipitate of insulin + zinc	7		Twice daily
Rapitard	Pig Beef	Solution and suspension	75% crystalline suspension 25% in solution	7	Actrapid MC	Once daily in mild diabetes
Monotard MC	Pig	Suspension	30% amorphous and 70% crystalline precipitated insulin + zinc	7	Actrapid MC Semitard MC	Usually daily
Lentard	Pig Beef	Suspension	30% amorphous and 70% crystalline precipated insulin + zinc	7	Actrapid MC Semitard MC	Usually daily

Protamine zinc insulin (PZI)†	Beef‡	Suspension	Amorphous precipitate of protamine, zinc and insulin	7	Actrapid MC	Once daily
Ultratard	Beef	Suspension	Crystalline precipitate insulin + zinc	7	Actrapid MC Semitard MC Lentard	Once daily

1. The monocomponent insulins can be mixed only with insulins of 'MC quality' if non-immunogenic properties are to be retained.
2. All insulin suspensions should be shaken immediately before filling the syringe and injecting.
3. Mixtures of insulin should be made in the syringe immediately prior to the injection.
4. The quantity of zinc added to all preparations is 2 mg/1000 U of insulin.
5. Lentard is a mixture of 30% Semilente (porcine) and 70% Ultratard (bovine), and its action is less intense but more prolonged than Monotard MC, because the latter is 10% porcine.

† These insulins are not manufactured by Novo, but are still currently used.
‡ Applicable to most manufacturers.
This table is reproduced with the kind permission of Novo Ltd., and incorporates their trade names.

Table 8.5   Insulin preparations classified by duration of action

Insulin	Time of action (h)		
	(a) Onset	(b) Peak effect	(c) Duration
Insulin injection ⎫ Neutral insulin injection ⎬ Neutral insulin injection MC ⎭	Quick ½–1	3–6	6–8
Insulin zinc suspension (amorphous)†	Fairly quick 1	3–6	12–14
Biphasic insulin injection	Fairly quick 1	4–10	24
Isophane insulin injection ⎫ Globin zinc insulin injection ⎪ Insulin zinc suspension ⎬‡ Insulin zinc suspension MC ⎪ Isophane insulin injection MC ⎭	Moderately delayed 2	6–12	24
Protamine zinc insulin injection ⎫ Insulin zinc suspension (crystalline) ⎬§	Delayed-onset 5–7	10–20	36

MC = monocomponent
The respective Novo nomenclature (see Table 8.5) is:
† Semilente or, the MC variety, Semitard
‡ Lente or Lentard which is 30 per cent Semilente and 70 per cent Ultratard
§ Ultralente or Ultratard which is the proinsulin-free preparation of Ultralente.
From Turner (1976). *Pharm. J.*, **217**, 583–4, by kind permission of the author and publishers.

   The ideal treatment of diabetes mellitus would be to inject a quick-acting insulin before each meal. This is not a practical solution, as most patients prefer only one injection a day. Thus the long-acting insulins are usually selected and these may achieve satisfactory control. If control is poor in the early part of the day, a short-acting insulin can also be given. Generally, if more than 60 units of a slow-acting insulin are required, it is necessary to alter the therapy to two short-acting insulins. Reference to Tables 8.4 and 8.5 provides a guide to the insulins, some of which are produced in combination. A combination of two compatible insulins which achieves good control in one patient may fail in another. It is important to know which insulins can be administered in the same syringe.
   In the future, it is probable that the monocomponent (MC) insulins only will be used, since these do not stimulate antibody formation. Lipodystrophy (see Plate 8.1), sometimes a distressing complication of the 'old' type of insulin, is also avoided by the use of the MC insulins. It must, however, be mentioned that the MC insulins have a more intense and shorter duration of action than the old types. Thus a patient who has been well controlled on the old type may require a smaller dose of the MC.

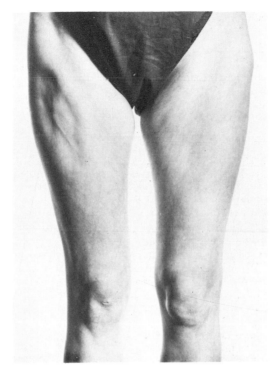

Plate 8.1   Marked lipodystrophy of the right thigh.

The most common insulins are available in concentrations of 20 units per ml, 40 units per ml, and 80 units per ml. In the United States and Canada insulin of 100 units per ml is used. The patient will often refer to the number of marks on his syringe as the number of units and this may mislead the inexperienced physician. It is obvious that if a patient changes from an insulin of 40 units per ml to one of 80 units per ml the volume of insulin in the syringe and consequently the numbers of marks will be halved, although the dose remains the same.

Diabetes and pregnancy

The potential diabetic tends to have large babies (over 4·5 kg), even though the diabetes does not become apparent until years later. In the diabetic mother complications such as toxaemia and hydramnios occur more frequently and the perinatal mortality is higher. The latter can be reduced appreciably by close co-operation between obstetrician, physician, and paediatrician. The mothers are admitted at the thirty-second week of pregnancy and their diabetes closely monitored. Frequent doses of short-acting insulin may be necessary in an attempt to keep the blood-glucose concentration at about 5·5 mmol/l (100 mg/100 ml) before meals. If delivery is too early the infant is endangered by prematurity and the respiratory distress syndrome. Probably the best procedure is to induce labour at the thirty-eighth week, since by this date the fetus has reached an adequate stage of maturity and further delay increases the risk of intrauterine death.

Glucagon

Excess

Glucagonoma

It has been observed that the plasma glucagon concentration is high in the ketoacidotic state of diabetes mellitus and may be responsible in part, for the acidosis. It has also been claimed that an excess of this hormone is a factor in the hyperglycaemia of uncontrolled diabetes mellitus, implying that a relative or absolute deficiency of insulin is not the sole cause. It is therefore of interest to note that recently a glucagonoma syndrome (hypersecretion of glucagon by a tumour) has been described.

Patients with glucagonoma are diabetic but they never develop ketoacidosis. There may be weight loss, a normochromic anaemia, and psychiatric disturbance. They are mostly postmenopausal women who display a peculiar rash, a necrolytic migratory erythema, usually over the lower abdomen, perineum, and thighs. The rash begins as an erythema, heals in the centre, and has a crusting edge. The surface is weeping in places and hyperpigmentation follows healing. Other features are circumoral cracking and glossitis. That the diabetes is so mild despite exceedingly high levels of glucagon suggests that this hormone is not the key factor in juvenile insulin-dependent diabetes. The diagnostic feature is a high level of plasma glucagon. Removal of the tumour results in the relief of symptoms and a cure of the diabetes.

9 Miscellaneous topics

This chapter considers a variety of topics which, excluding the prostaglandins, appear to be related by the APUD theory. This concept is therefore considered in the first section. The subjects discussed in this chapter are presented in the following order:

1. The theory of APUD cells and apudoma
2. Ectopic secretion (production of hormones by non-endocrine tumours)
3. Multiple endocrine adenomatosis
4. Tumour of δ-cells of the pancreatic islets
5. 5-Hydroxytryptamine (serotonin) and carcinoids
6. Prostaglandins

The APUD concept and apudoma

During the course of fetal development, certain neuroectodermal cells migrate from the central nervous system to different parts of the body, but particularly to the region derived embryologically from the upper part of the alimentary canal. These migratory cells share a number of cytochemical and ultrastructural characteristics. For example they contain amines, they have the capacity to assimilate amine precursors, and they contain amine acid decarboxylase. These features have led to such cells being referred to collectively as APUD cells (amine content and/or *A*mine *P*recursor *U*ptake and *D*ecarboxylation) cells. It is claimed that these cells may give rise to a wide range of endocrine cells such as the C-cells of the thyroid, the α-, β-, and δ-cells of the pancreatic islets, the cells of the pars distalis, and the disseminated hormone-secretory cells of the alimentary tract. It is believed that carcinoids which secrete 5-hydroxytryptamine (5-HT) and other substances can be considered as tumours of the APUD cell system. A generalized term for all types of tumour of this system is apudoma. The apudoma may secrete an excess of the polypeptide (hormone) appropriate to the cell which has become neoplastic (orthoendocrine syndrome). Alternatively the neoplastic cells may become dedifferentiated (possibly by derepression) and secrete an inappropriate hormone, or hormones (paraendocrine syndrome). This could account for the ectopic hormone syndrome. Another interesting aspect of this theory is that it offers an explanation for the syndrome of multiple endocrine adenomatosis which is characterized by the presence of tumours occurring in several endocrine glands. This concept is ingenious but it remains to be proved that, for example, the cells which gives rise to an oat-cell carcinoma when it secretes an ectopic hormone are an apudoma.

Ectopic secretion (production of hormones by non-endocrine tumours)

It is common for a tumour of an endocrine gland to secrete the hormone which is normally produced by the healthy gland; however the hormone is usually secreted in excess and does not respond to the normal control mechanisms. If the affected gland normally produces several different hormones, the tumour may produce only one of these or it may produce several, perhaps in abnormal proportions; sometimes it may even secrete excessive amounts of a hormone precursor. This suggests that the synthesis pathways in tumour cells may differ from those in normal endocrine cells. Endocrine tumours generally produce the appropriate hormones, even though they may do so in inappropriate ways and in inappropriate amounts.

Of greater biological interest is the comparatively recent recognition that hormones are secreted by many tumours which arise in organs not normally associated with endocrine activity. These tumours of non-endocrine tissue, which are frequently malignant, may induce the clinical syndrome which is similar to that of hypersecretion of the appropriate endocrine gland. When this occurs it is usually referred to as ectopic secretion, as the hormone is being secreted from an abnormal site. There is the added complexity that a tumour of an endocrine gland may secrete a 'foreign' hormone (i.e. one that in the normal state is not secreted by that gland); this secretion is also referred to as ectopic.

For some years it has been realized that tumours may produce metabolic effects quite out of proportion to their size. For example, one of the commonest metabolic disturbances produced by malignant tumours is hypercalcaemia. In many cases this is due to skeletal metastases producing local areas of bone lysis with the consequent liberation of excess calcium into the circulation. There is no doubt, however, that occasionally hypercalcaemia may be produced by tumours in the absence of metastases in bone. The tumour is therefore presumably liberating some calcium mobilizing substance into the circulation. It has been shown that in a proportion of such cases, although not in all, the substance is parathormone, which appears to be identical with normal parathormone originating from the parathyroid glands. Parathormone secretion seems to be a feature of squamous cell carcinoma of the lung (ectopic secretion). In non-metastatic tumours producing hypercalcaemia in which it has been impossible to detect parathyroid hormone production, it has been suggested that prostaglandins or vitamin D-like steroids may be responsible, but these have not yet been demonstrated unequivocally.

The 'ectopic ACTH (corticotrophin) syndrome', one of the commoner examples of such a disorder, has been extensively studied. This syndrome is usually associated with oat-cell carcinoma of the lung, and is due to increased circulating levels of cortisol as a result of stimulation of the adrenal cortex by the ectopically secreted corticotrophin. Despite this, however, patients with ectopic corticotrophin secretion due to oat-cell carcinoma rarely develop the typical picture of Cushing's syndrome (Chapter 4), perhaps because so few of them survive for a sufficient period of time. The most striking features of this condition are usually hypokalaemic alkalosis and profound muscular weakness. In those instances when the ectopic corticotrophin is produced by tumours such as thymomas or carcinoids, which may be non-malignant, the clinical picture may be that of classical Cushing's syndrome; the differential diagnosis from corticotrophin hypersecretion by the adenohypophysis may then be extremely difficult. Originally this diagnosis in some patients was revealed only when treatment directed at the adenohypophysis failed to produce any alteration in the course of the Cushing's syndrome. Although the ectopic corticotrophin syndrome is only clinically apparent in about 3 per cent of cases with oat-cell carcinoma of the lung, as many as 50 per cent of cases show some disturbance of cortisol secretion and regulation which are detectable biochemically. Recent evidence suggests that increased levels of corticotrophin may in fact occur in all oat-cell or carcinoid tumours and, still more interestingly, increased corticotrophin levels have been found in areas of lung tissue which were not involved by the tumour. Although immunoactivity is consistently higher than bioactivity, the levels are found to be elevated by both techniques. Nevertheless, not all such patients show overt signs of the ectopic corticotrophin syndrome.

Another relatively common metabolic abnormality associated with oat-cell carcinomas of the lung is hyponatraemia, now recognized to be due in many instances to the ectopic secretion of vasopressin. If the hyponatraemia is due to an excess of vasopressin the typical water retention syndrome which is described in the section on inappropriate secretion of vasopressin (Chapter 2) is seen.

The recognition that tumours may secrete a comparatively wide range of hormones has naturally led to a great deal of speculation on how this might arise. The most probable explanation appears to be that when a cell becomes neoplastic, sections of the gene which are normally repressed may become available for transcription. This explains why only polypeptide hormones have so far been conclusively shown to be produced ectopically. The production of a steroid, for instance, would require a complex enzymic pathway to be developed, which seems an extremely improbable consequence of random derepression. As it is debatable whether prostaglandins or vitamin D steroids can be synthesized, the theory is still tenable. However, one problem with the derepression theory is that it does not explain why certain types of tumour preferentially secrete particular hormones. If derepression were random one might expect the type of hormones produced to be random, apart from its being polypeptide in structure.

A possible explanation for this specificity of hormone production by tumours is given by the theory that the cells which produce such hormones when they undergo neoplastic change have a common embryological derivation, namely that they are APUD cells. Whatever may ultimately prove to be the correct explanation, it is clear that the ectopic production of hormones by tumours arising in non-endocrine tissues is a fascinating field of study. Not only is it possibly a valuable insight into the nature of the neoplastic process, but the hormones secreted may act as 'tumour markers', permitting early diagnosis perhaps even before any pathological change can be detected; furthermore the plasma hormone concentration may be used to monitor therapy and to assess its effectiveness. In this connection it must be remembered that not all the peptides produced by tumours are hormones, but that others such as carcino-embryonic antigen, α-feto protein, and the Regan isoenzyme of alkaline phosphatase may have similar significance.

Multiple endocrine adenomatosis

Multiple endocrine adenomatosis is a condition which involves the hyperfunction of more than one endocrine gland. It could be explained by the APUD theory, as example of multiple apudomas. The disorder is inherited as an autosomal dominant gene, but may occur sporadically. The particular glands involved and the nature of the hyperfunction of each differ, such that there is considerable variation in the expression and character of the disease. Two main types of multiple endocrine adenomatosis can be distinguished on the basis that various glands are more commonly involved together. Hyperparathyroidism is the only feature common to the two types. Any combination of disorder within each type may occur (see Table 9.1).

Table 9.1   Multiple endocrine adenomatosis

Type I
1. Gastrin excess (Zollinger–Ellison syndrome)
2. Insulin excess
3. Chromophobe adenoma
4. Acromegaly
5. Diffuse hyperplasia, or adenoma of the parathyroid
6. Carcinoid (occasional)
7. Associated conditions—multiple lipomata

Type II
1. Phaeochromocytoma (often bilateral)
2. Medullary thyroid carcinoma (bilateral)
3. Parathyroid (diffuse hyperplasia)
4. Cushing's disease (rare)
5. Associated conditions—neuromata; neurofibromata

Tumour of δ-cells of the pancreatic islets

The only known function of the δ-cells is to secrete gastrin; the role of somastatin is uncertain (see Chapter 8). The syndrome described by Zollinger–Ellison in 1955 is associated with tumour of the δ-cells, but encompasses a wider field than tumour of the δ-cells alone.

The original description of the Zollinger–Ellison syndrome was that of a fulminating, sometimes fatal, peptic ulceration with multiple ulcers in atypical sites, such as the jejunum. The ulceration is usually associated with massive hypersecretion of gastric acid, although this is not invariable. It was initially considered to be a 'gastrin-secreting non-β islet cell tumour', but a gastrin-secreting tumour may arise in the duodenal wall. Thus reference is made to a gastrinoma in order to include both sites.

The tumours are often small and multiple. In 60 per cent of cases they are malignant while 30 per cent have multiple benign tumours, and in 10 per cent there is a diffuse hyperlasia of the gastrin-secreting pancreatic δ-islet cells. Although these tumours secrete the gastrointestinal polypeptide hormone gastrin, they may, on some occasions, also secrete a combination of hormones such as corticotrophin, MSH, and insulin (ectopic secretion). These tumours or hyperplastic islets may form part of the multiple endocrine adenomatosis syndrome (MEA).

Microscopically these tumours are well differentiated with trabeculae or sheets of cells, very similar to carcinoid tumours. The diagnosis is confirmed by extracting gastrin from the tumour or by demonstrating the presence of gastrin in the tumour by immunofluorescence using a gastrin-specific antibody labelled with fluorescein.

The condition is first suspected when a patient develops symptoms suggesting a recurrent peptic ulcer after conventionally adequate surgery. In such cases the pain experienced is typically severe and relentless. Repeated life-threatening haemorrhages or perforation are common occurrences, often within days or weeks of surgery. Physical examination may show a scar from previous gastric surgery. Rarely a mass is palpable in the epigastrium or there may be hepatomegaly due to multiple small hepatic metastases.

INVESTIGATIONS:

1. In a patient with an intact stomach prior to surgery the 12-h overnight gastric acid secretion is raised (greater than 100 mmol HCl/12 h), as is the basal acid secretion (greater than 15 mmol/h). The ratio of basal acid output (BAO) to maximal acid output (MAO) following the injection of pentagastrin is high (>0.6). Any partially gastrectomized patient with a basal secretion greater than 5 mmol/h warrants further investigation.

2. Serum gastrin, whether measured by biological or radio-immunological methods, is usually elevated. Radio-immunoassay is now the common method used and, in the absence of pyloric stenosis, levels above 500 μg/l are usually regarded as diagnostic depending on individual laboratories. Levels over 200 μg/l are indicative of the syndrome, especially if associated with gastric hypersecretion. However hypergastrinaemia alone is not necessarily diagnostic, since gastrin levels may be high in conditions such as pernicious anaemia (with achlorhydria), following vagotomy after gastric resection with retained gastric antrum, in renal failure, and in anephric patients on chronic haemodialysis. This is not an exhaustive list and each case must be carefully studied. In order to distinguish gastrinoma from other causes of hypergastrinaemia, stimulatory tests are employed. The normal gastric antral mucosa secretes in response to food whereas a tumour does not. Conversely a gastrinoma is highly sensitive to infusions of calcium or secretin, inducing enhanced levels of gastrin, whereas the normal stomach (including the patient with a duodenal ulcer) shows little response or even a decrease in gastrin levels.

3. Radiological studies of the upper gastrointestinal tract show peptic ulceration, often in atypical sites, with coarse gastric folds, a dilated duodenum and jejunum, and blunted valvulae conniventes.

4. Special investigations: selective arteriography, pancreatic isotope scanning, and ultrasonography are of limited use in localizing the tumours due to their small size.

Finally, the diagnosis may be made by laparotomy when a pancreatic mass or hepatic metastases are found. Unfortunately, if there are small multiple tumours, they are often not palpable.

TREATMENT: The only effective standard treatment until recently was a total gastrectomy. This removes the target organ, without affecting the secretion of gastrin. Less drastic surgery has a high postoperative mortality resulting from recurrent ulceration, perforation, and haemorrhage. Only rarely is it possible to resect an isolated gastrinoma and, as there may be other undetected tumours or metastases, such a procedure without an additional total gastrectomy is unwise. The prognosis after total gastrectomy is good and even in the presence of a malignant tumour it is not unusual for patients to live 10–15 years with multiple hepatic metastases together with extremely high circulating gastrin levels. Recently the introduction of cimetidine, a receptor blocker which inhibits the histamine releasing action of gastrin, has made conservative treatment feasible. This drug by blocking the action of histamine on the parietal cell decreases gastric acid secretion, even in the presence of the powerful stimulation by raised gastrin levels. Only a few patients with the syndrome have been treated with this drug and it remains to be established whether long-term therapy will be effective.

5-Hydroxytryptamine (serotonin) and carcinoids

5-Hydroxytryptamine

In mammals 5-hydroxytryptamine (5-HT) is present mainly in the enterochromaffin cells of the gastrointestinal tract. It is also present in small amounts in platelets and in the central nervous system. Although not present in human mast cells, it has been found in mast cell tumours of man. It is accepted that the brain controls the secretion of hypothalamic hormones/factors, through neural connections, and this effect is mediated by neurotransmitters which are the monamines, dopamine, noradrenalin, and 5-HT. The latter stimulates the secretion of PIF (prolactin inhibiting factor) and GHRF (growth hormone releasing factor). Certain tumours (carcinoid) of enterochromaffin or related cells may develop in the gastrointestinal tract (frequently the terminal ileum) or respiratory tract. The clinical importance of 5-HT stems from the fact that carcinoids secrete excessive quantities of this substance, in addition to a precursor substance, active polypeptides, and/or prostaglandins.

Tryptophan is converted into 5-hydroxytryptophan by means of the enzyme tryptophan hydroxylase which is present in all carcinoid tumours. From 5-hydroxytryptophan, 5-HT is formed. The degradation of 5-HT occurs mainly in the liver where it is converted to 5-hydroxyindole acetaldehyde by the enzyme monoaminoxidase (MAO). This acetaldehyde is then rapidly converted to the excretory product 5-hydroxyindole acetic acid (5-HIAA) by aldehyde dehydrogenase.

Carcinoids

This term is used for all tumours which develop from argentaffin cells, usually of the intestinal mucosa (argentaffinoma, staining with silver or chromium compounds). These can also be considered as apudomas. The usual site of the tumour is such that its secretion flows to the liver where inactivation occurs. Symptoms and signs are not present until metastases form into this organ.

However, carcinoid tumours of the bronchus (or rarely the gonads) can release humoral substances directly into the systemic circulation to induce effects before reaching the liver. The typical clinical picture is of a patient with abdominal discomfort and diarrhoea; frequently these are the most distressing features. Telangiectasia develops in the skin and marked, bright red flushes over the face and chest may occur spontaneously or in response to stress. Bronchoconstriction is less commonly observed. In the cardiovascular system there may be stenosis or incompetence of the pulmonary or tricuspid valves due to collagenous deposits, which may lead to heart failure. Certain of these changes are associated with carcinoids at special sites. For example, gastric carcinoids are usually associated with flushes, but diarrhoea and heart lesions occur less frequently; carcinoid tumours of the bronchus are frequently associated with vomiting, diarrhoea, and severe bronchoconstriction. Of all these changes 5-HT can only be accepted as being responsible for the diarrhoea and gastrointestinal malabsorption. Other substances secreted such as bradykinin and possibly prostaglandins could be responsible for the other clinical manifestations.

If the tumour is very large it may metabolize a large proportion of available tryptophan, thus diverting it from niacin and protein formation. It is claimed that this causes the occasional occurrence of pellagra and hypoalbuminaemia in these patients.

Diagnosis of the carcinoid tumour depends on an increased excretion of 5-HIAA, although it is important to note that certain foods (for example walnuts and bananas) contain enough 5-HT to produce an abnormally elevated urinary excretion of 5-HIAA after ingestion.

The treatment of this condition is if possible surgical removal of the tumour. If this is not possible or if secondary deposits have occurred, drug therapy is employed. If alimentary canal symptoms are the major complaint, anti-serotonin agents may be used, either as competitive inhibitors (methysergide) or inhibitors of synthesis (*p*-chlorophenylalanine). Attacks of flushes may be reduced in frequency with α-adrenergic blocker (phenoxybenzamine 10 mg t.d.s.). It must be emphasized that nutrition must be maintained and vitamin supplements given (in particular niacin). Steroid therapy induces a marked improvement in patients with bronchoconstriction.

Prostaglandins

Initially it was observed that human semen, as well as extracts of sheep vesicular glands, possessed the property of stimulating isolated intestinal and uterine smooth muscle. Within a few years it was established that the pharmacological effects of human semen were due to a completely new substance referred to as 'prostaglandin' in the mistaken belief that it was secreted by the prostate gland. However, it is now known that the prostaglandins of human seminal fluid originate in the seminal vesicles.

Originally, two compounds, one soluble in ether and the other in phosphate buffer, were isolated. The ether-soluble substance was called prostaglandin E (PGE) and the other, which was soluble in phosphate buffer (in Swedish, phosphate is spelt with an F) was called prostaglandin F (PGF). Other prostaglandins are listed alphabetically in the order in which they are discovered;

the subsequent naturally occurring prostaglandin has therefore been named PGA (medullin).

These substances are a group of biologically active 20-carbon hydroxy fatty acids with a cyclopentane ring and two chains. Of importance to obstetrics are the PGEs and PGFs, the difference in the structure between these two groups being in the cyclopentane (5-carbon) ring. The number of unsaturated carbon bonds in the chain is donated by a subscript numeral. Thus, PGE_1 has one double bond in the side chain whereas PGE_2 has two double bonds. The subscript α or β denotes the position of a hydroxyl group in position 9, as to whether it is below or above the molecular plane. Two prostaglandins, dinoprostone (PGE_2, Prostin E_2—Upjohn) and dinoprost (PGF_2 Prostin F_2—Upjohn) are now marketed in Britain. The exact role of prostaglandins in the control of physiological processes has yet to be clarified.

Biosynthesis and catabolism

Most cells are capable of synthesizing prostaglandins from essential fatty acid precursors *in vivo*, especially from arachidonic acid which is the most abundant free fatty acid in the body. Unlike many other biologically active substances, prostaglandins are formed immediately prior to their release and are therefore not stored in the body. A variety of stimuli are capable of releasing prostaglandins following the activation of phospholipase A which leads to the release of precursors from cellular phospholipid stores. Synthesis of the primary prostaglandins is accomplished in stepwise manner by a complex microsomal enzyme system referred to as 'prostaglandin synthetase'. Non-steroidal anti-inflammatory agents such as aspirin and indomethacin act by inhibiting prostaglandin synthesis.

Prostaglandins E_2 and F_2 are very rapidly metabolized in the kidneys, lungs, and liver. The measurement of levels of metabolites which are more stable may therefore contribute to an appreciation of the physiological role of prostaglandins in the body. Metabolism of prostaglandins usually results in the curtailment of their activity. The 13,14-dihydro derivative of PGF_2, however, has an oxytocic activity which approaches that of its parent compound and probably contributes to the uterine stimulation observed during intravenous infusion of PGF_2.

Physiological role

Prostaglandins probably act as 'local hormones', i.e. they are produced for a local action rather than being produced at one site and then acting some distance away from it. Most interest has been attached to the possible involvement of prostaglandins in reproductive physiology. The presence of prostaglandin in very high concentration in semen, together with the observation that prostaglandins are substantially absorbed by the vagina have encouraged speculation that prostaglandins facilitate conception during coitus. Furthermore, low levels of prostaglandins in the semen have been associated with infertility in humans (although prostaglandins are sparse or even absent in the semen of other species). Their exact role in male fertility must therefore still be regarded as speculative.

In many laboratory and farm animals PGF_2 released from the uterus has been identified as a luteolytic factor, but no clear influence of PGF_2 on the regression of the human corpus luteum has yet been demonstrated. With regard to pregnancy, as prostaglandin levels rise sharply in the amniotic fluid at term, it is thought that they may play a role in parturition. It would then be possible to explain the observation that the intake of large amounts of aspirin in pregnancy results in a prolongation of the second stage of labour.

In addition, prostaglandins have been implicated as factors regulating tone in many smooth muscles, perhaps by being partly responsible for the auto-regulation of renal blood-flow and the regulation of blood-pressure. There is evidence that prostaglandins are in part responsible for the inflammatory response and for the hyperpyrexia observed in some infections. It has been suggested that the beneficial effects of aspirin and indomethacin are achieved by their inhibitory action on prostaglandin synthesis.

It has also been proposed that prostaglandins play a role at the cellular level by modulating the effects of other hormones. Trophic hormones such as LH, corticotrophin, and thyrotrophin interact with membrane receptors which lead to an increase in prostaglandin synthetase and prostaglandin production. The prostaglandins in turn may activate membrane adenyl cyclase, possibly through a specific prostaglandin receptor. The resultant increase in cyclic AMP (adenosine $3',5'$-monophosphate) would then produce its action on cell function (see Chapter 10). The therapeutic applications of prostaglandins are at present restricted to the use of PGE_2 and PGF_2 in the induction of labour or abortion.

Originally it was believed that this family of substances was of fundamental importance in implementing the effects of hormones by acting as intracellular second messengers. In addition, these substances were regarded as important local hormones (e.g. altering blood-flow). Unfortunately the initial expectations were unfulfilled and the study of the prostaglandins has not yet provided a significant insight into the basic physiological action of hormones and whether they are important as local hormones is debatable.

10 Hormonal mechanisms of action at the cellular level

The precise way in which a particular hormone can exert a specific effect on its target cell is an intriguing problem which at present is only partly understood. Originally it was believed that each hormone exerted its characteristic effect through an individual action. Thus vasopressin influenced water reabsorption by a process which was not comparable with that of adrenalin on glycogenolysis in the liver. It now appears that the hormonal mechanisms of action have certain common components and that specificity is dependent on the type of receptor to which the hormone is bound. In this chapter, first the hormone receptor theory of specificity will be briefly considered, and then the general theories of hormone action.

The receptor theory

The characteristic actions of a hormone depend on its 'recognition' by the target cell. This recognition is therefore a property of the cell and must involve receptors which are specific for that hormone. Thus the follicular cells of the thyroid have receptor molecules which are specific for thyrotrophin molecules from the adenohypophysis; the myoepithelial cells of the breasts have specific receptors for oxytocin; etc. The recognition between receptor and hormone molecules can be compared to the way in which a key fits a lock. For any particular lock there is only one key which will fit it perfectly. This 'lock and key' principle is shown in Fig 10.1. Pursuing the analogy further, it is possible that the sharing of actions to varying degrees between different hormones is comparable with the observation that a slightly different key may with persuasion 'force the lock'. For example oxytocin and vasopressin, the two octapeptides from the neurohypophysis which have similar chemical structures

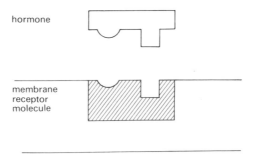

hormone

membrane
receptor
molecule

Fig.10.1   The 'lock and key' principle of hormone–receptor interaction.

(differing only in the nature of two of the amino acids), both have their own distinct actions, but these are nevertheless shared to a small degree. Oxytocin therefore has some antidiuretic activity, while vasopressin can stimulate uterine contraction.

Cellular recognition by receptor molecules can take place at two general sites in the cell: at the plasma membranes or inside the cell. The majority of protein, peptide, or amine hormones do not have to enter the cell to exert their various effects. Insulin is a prime example of such a hormone, for it can be bound to very large molecules forming complexes which can not possibly penetrate the cell membrane and yet it still exerts its various effects on the transport of molecules across the membrane as well as influencing particular enzyme systems within the cell. The manner in which insulin and other hormones can alter intracellular mechanisms without entering the cytoplasm may be explained on the basis of another general theory: the theory of 'second messengers' which will be considered later in the chapter.

Many hormones, especially steroids can penetrate the plasma membranes so that recognition occurs somewhere within the target cells themselves. Specificity is therefore determined after the hormone has entered the cells by the presence of intracellular receptor molecules. When the appropriate hormones are applied to the target cells the observed increase in intracellular RNA is not immediate. This and other experimental evidence has led to the theory that these hormones form complexes with their specific receptors, and that these complexes often act by stimulating protein synthesis at the nuclear level or subsequently by enhancing protein synthesis in the cytoplasm.

General theories of hormone action

There are three general theories by which a hormone can exert its effects on its specific target cells (a) by direct membrane effects; (b) by intracellular effects through the activation of a 'second messenger'; (c) by direct intracellular effects on protein synthesis. While these three general theories form a convenient system for categorizing hormones, it must be emphasized that a hormone can influence any combination of these mechanisms. In addition some hormones have not so far been shown to act by any of these mechanisms, and therefore it must be remembered that other modes of action probably exist and remain to be discovered.

1. Direct membrane effects

A hormone can have a direct effect on the permeability of plasma membranes such that transport characteristics for particular molecules are altered. This could result from the interaction between hormone and specific membrane receptor such that the structure of the membrane itself is altered (e.g. by the opening up of pores), by influencing the activity of some form of carrier molecule (e.g by altering its structure thereby increasing its affinity for the particular salute being transported) or by activating or influencing an active pump mechanism.

While the various membrane effects of insulin on the transport of monosaccharides such as glucose, the transport of amino acids, and the maintenance

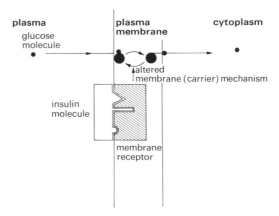

Fig.10.2 Diagram illustrating how insulin could react with its receptor and alter the facilitated transport mechanism for glucose.

of a high intracellular potassium ion concentration can be explained in terms of altered membrane characteristics due to the binding which occurs on that membrane between insulin and its receptor (see Fig. 10.2), it is difficult to account for the changes in enzymatic activity within the cell itself. On theory to account for this intracellular effect of insulin is based on the assumption that normally the cell membrane is highly permeable to glucose and an active pump mechanism is necessary to continually extrude the glucose (cf. sodium pump). Insulin could, by inhibiting this pump mechanism, increase the intracellular glucose concentration. Furthermore, the surplus 'energy' released by inhibiting the activity of the pump could be diverted to those intracellular processes which result in the enzymatic changes associated with the effects of insulin (Fig. 10.3). This theory is based upon the observation that anoxia and certain metabolic inhibitors appear to mimic the effect of insulin upon the cellular entry of glucose. However many of the metabolic consequences appear to differ and this theory is at present considered unlikely.

2. Intracellular second messenger activation theory

Those hormones (first messengers) which react with plasma membrane receptors and yet exert intracellular actions could activate cytoplasmic systems which then act as 'second messengers'. This second messenger system can then initiate the various intracellular effects which characterize the hormone, either by influencing previously existing enzyme systems or by stimulating the synthesis of new protein. Some membrane effects associated with hormones could in fact be due to (and probably are) the activation of intracellular messenger systems, involved in the formation of enzymes which can influence the cytoplasmic surface of the cell membrane (see Fig. 10.4).

Various 'second messengers' have been proposed including prostaglandins, intracellular calcium, ions, cyclic AMP (cyclic adenosine 3′,5′-monophosphate, cAMP) and cyclic GMP (cyclic guanosine 3′,5′-

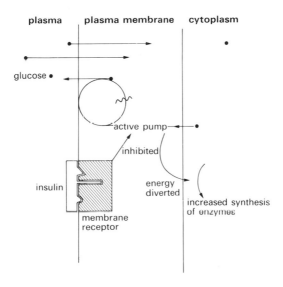

Fig.10.3 Diagram illustrating how insulin could produce its membrane and intracellular effects by inhibiting a postulated active glucose pump.

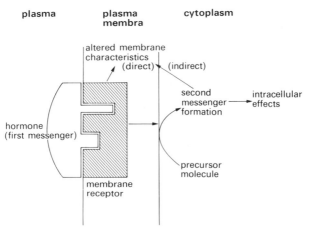

Fig.10.4 Diagram illustrating how the formation of a second messenger could result in the indirect alteration of membrane characteristics.

monophosphate, cGMP). Of these various second messengers, one in particular, cyclic cAMP, has received considerable attention and therefore will be briefly discussed.

In the presence of magnesium or manganese ions this cyclic nucleotide is formed from adenosine triphosphate (ATP) by the action of an enzyme, which in mammalian cells is mainly membrane-bound, called adenyl cyclase. Cyclic AMP then activates various enzymes called protein kinases by catalysing the transfer of the terminal phosphate of ATP to the kinase. These activated protein kinases may then induce the intracellular effects associated with the various first messenger hormones. Cyclic AMP is degraded by hydrolysis to 5'-adenosine monophosphate (5'AMP) this reaction being catalysed by phosphodiesterase enzyme.

The best-known action of cyclic AMP was shown by Sutherland and Hall in 1958. Their experiments indicated that the formation of this cyclic nucleotide was the intermediate step between the hormone adrenalin and its glycogenolytic action in hepatic tissue. The activation of the protein kinase by cyclic AMP resulted in the subsequent activation of phosphorylase which is the enzyme involved in splitting glycogen down to glucose 1-phosphate, resulting ultimately in an increased plasma concentration of glucose (see Fig. 10.5).

Some of the actions of other hormones, in addition to adrenalin, also appear to coincide with increases in intracellular cyclic AMP concentrations. However great care must be taken before it is assumed that the actions of a

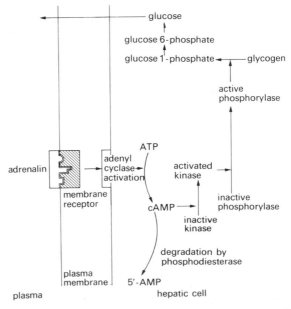

Fig.10.5   Diagram illustrating how the activation of cyclic AMP by the interaction of adrenalin with its receptor results in glycogenolysis in the liver.

particular hormone are always due to its induction of cyclic AMP. For example, several hormones which are known to increase cyclic AMP concentrations in some cell systems (namely catecholamines, vasopressin, oxytocin, and angiotensin II) can produce effects in other cells which are not related to changes in intracellular levels of this cyclic nucleotide. In any particular hormone-target cell system under investigation, certain criteria should always be satisfied before cyclic AMP is accepted as the second messenger. First, the hormone should be capable of stimulating adenyl cyclase activity in a cell-free system; secondly, the hormone should increase the cyclic AMP concentration in an intact cell system in a manner compatible with the effects of the hormone in that particular tissue (with respect to time–course and dose–response relationships); and thirdly, that cyclic AMP should be able to reproduce the effects of the hormone when added to an intact cell system. Even if these criteria are satisfied one cannot conclude that cyclic AMP is involved in all the actions of the hormone being investigated, since other second messenger systems can also be stimulated by that same hormone.

Some of the hormones which have so far been shown to involve cyclic AMP in at least one of their actions are listed in Table 10.1.

Table 10.1 Some hormones which have been shown to involve the cyclic AMP in the determination of at least one of their actions.

Hormones	Target tissues
Adrenalin	Many
Vasopressin	Toad bladder, kidney
Corticotrophin	Adrenal cortex
LH	Ovary, corpus luteum, testis
Glucagon	Liver, fat
Parathormone	Kidney, bone

Another aspect of the 'second messenger' concept is the possibility that, in some instances at least, it acts only as an intermediate messenger in the transfer of information reaching the cell to the activation of intracellular processes, and that further messenger systems are involved. For example, increase osteoclastic activity may be induced by the *cytoplasmic* calcium ions concentration which is raised by the actions of parathormone. This hormonal effect may be partly induced by the stimulation of cyclic AMP which increases the efflux of calcium ions from the mitochondrial stores, and to a direct action by parathormone on the osteoclastic cell membrane to increase the net influx of calcium into the cell. The raised cytoplasmic calcium ions concentration is then believed to act as another messenger by stimulating the synthesis of enzymes and possible the rupturing of lysosomes. These enzymes may induce osteoclastic activity which increases the reabsorption of the calcium matrix. This accounts for one of the actions of parathormone on bone (see Chapter 7). Indeed, a close relationship between calcium ions and cyclic AMP activity has also been suggested, implying that the regulation of many hormonal effects is undoubtedly a complex procedure involving various different factors.

3. Intracellular effects of hormones on protein synthesis

The various metabolic processes which regulate the functions of a cell are controlled by enzymes. These enzymes consist of genetically determined arrangements of amino acids, the codes for which reside in the genes of nuclear chromosomes. As mentioned previously, steroid hormones are capable of penetrating the plasma membranes of cells to combine with their specific cytoplasmic receptors. Some of the complexes thus formed appear to be able to influence protein synthesis at the nuclear level, which suggests that they activate particular gene sequences. One mechanism which has been suggested for this action is that the hormone–receptor complex can combine with a specific regulator gene, whose role normally is to repress the activity of adjacent genes which are involved in the synthesis of a particular protein. Genes consist of deoxyribonucleic acid molecules (DNA). Jacob and Monod (1959) suggested that the repressor gene inhibits the adjacent operator gene which itself controls the activity of the adjacent structural genes. Removal of the influence of the repressor gene (by combination with the hormone–receptor complex) would liberate the operator gene so that the structural genes would be activated. This activation process would result in the synthesis of ribonucleic acid molecules (RNA). Some of these RNA molecules then act as messengers (mRNA) for the new protein code, and move out of the cell nucleus to the cytoplasmic ribosomes (RNA) where they become attached in order to ensure that the amino acids are linked in the correct sequence for the required protein to be synthesized. Other RNA molecules (transfer RNA, tRNA) then transfer the various amino acids to the ribosomes with the consequent synthesis of the new, specific protein (Fig. 10.6).

There are two stages in the synthesis of protein that can be influenced by hormones or their complexes: (1) the transcription of the code from DNA to mRNA and (2) the translation of the mRNA code to the synthesis of the protein on the ribosomes. Steroid hormones such as cortisol and oestrogen stimulate protein (enzyme) synthesis mainly at the transcription stage since their effects can be largely blocked by actinomycin D which irreversibly combines with the DNA molecules. The protein synthesis induced by T_4 and T_3 and insulin are believed in part also to act at the transcription stage. The effects of other hormones which stimulate cellular protein synthesis are not completely blocked by actinomycin D, but are by puromycin which inhibits the translation stage. These hormones, such as somatotrophin, are therefore assumed to stimulate the translation stage possibly by increasing the rate at which tRNA takes up amino acids.

Finally, protein synthesis can in addition be influenced by other, less direct, mechanisms. For example, protein synthesis requires energy in the form of ATP and other nucleoside triphosphates, and hence any alterations in energy supply could be considered to be a crude, unspecific form of regulation. The availability of amino acids is similarly a potential limiting factor to the process, and hormones such as insulin which influence amino acid transport across the plasma membrane could also influence protein synthesis through this mechanism.

(a)

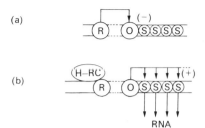

(b)

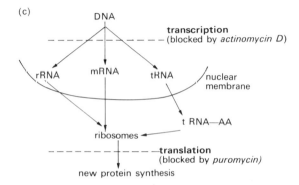

Fig.10.6 The inhibition of the operator gene (O) by the repressor gene (R) in a nuclear chromo-some (a) can be removed by the combination of the repressor gene with the hormone–receptor complex (H-RC). The operator gene can then activate the structural genes (S) with the consequent formation of various types of RNA (b).

(c) Shows the transcription stage which results in the formation of ribosomal RNA (rRNA), messenger RNA (mRNA) and transfer RNA (tRNA) in the nucleus. The translation stage is when the individual amino acids are united in the correct sequence for the new protein synthesis on the cytoplasmic ribosomes.

Summary

Once a hormone has been recognized by its target cell by combining with its specific receptor it acts on cellular processes through one or more of three principal mechanisms; (1) by altering plasma membrane permeability charac-teristics; (2) by activating 'second' and even 'third' messenger systems inside the cell which can then alter cellular metabolism; (3) by stimulating protein synthesis directly, either at the transcription or at the translation stages.

The most investigated 'second messenger' system at present is the adenyl-cyclase (cAMP) system, although the importance of the intracellular Ca^{2+} concentration as a messenger is now realized. It must nevertheless be appre-ciated that our knowledge of the intracellular mechanisms of hormonal action is still far from complete.

11 Acute endocrine emergencies

In this chapter it is possible only to provide guidelines by which the student may be able to establish the identity of an underlying endocrine disorder. The conditions discussed in this chapter are given in Table 11.1.

Table 11.1 Acute endocrine emergencies

1. Diabetes mellitus:
   a. hyperglycaemia with ketoacidosis
   b. hyperglycaemia without ketoacidosis, (hyperosmolar)
   c. hyperglycaemia with lactic acidosis
2. Hypoglycaemia
3. Myxoedema coma
4. Hypopituitary coma
5. Addisonian crisis
6. Hypocalcaemia
7. Hypercalcaemia
8. Thyroid crisis
9. Hypertensive crisis in phaeochromocytoma

The importance of a previous 'history' and careful clinical examination cannot be overemphasized. Problems arise when the patient is unconscious and the history has to be obtained from a relative. On clinical examination the following observations are of value:

1. The state of consciousness (drowsiness, stupor, coma)
2. The facial appearance and the odour of the breath
3. The state of hydration, presence of sweating, colour of mucous membranes
4. The rate and character of respiration, pulse-rate and blood-pressure
5. The temperature using a low-reading thermometer
6. The colour and texture of the skin, the distribution of facial and body hair
7. The reflexes, visual fields, and optic fundi
8. Examination of the urine

As the treatment of an acute endocrine emergency is urgent, it is not possible to wait for biochemical confirmation of the clinical diagnosis. Nevertheless such tests are required, since errors of diagnosis may occur; in addition they provide a guideline for further therapy.

In clinical practice diabetic coma is an imprecise definition. Many would accept that the distinction between diabetic coma and pre-coma is vague and hence of no value. The problem is to define that condition in which a patient with diabetes mellitus requires urgent therapy to correct the metabolic disorder. Provided a definition of the term is given, errors of semantics are avoided. In this book 'diabetic coma', a rare condition, is applied to those patients with such severe hyperglycaemia and marked dehydration that they require urgent treatment; frequently these patients show some disturbance of consciousness. Three separate varieties are described: hyperglycaemia with ketoacidosis (the commonest variety), hyperglycaemia without ketoacidosis (hyperosmolar), and hyperglycaemia with lactic acidosis. It is accepted that there is some overlap between ketotic hyperglycaemia and the non-ketotic variety. Furthermore, it is appreciated that the plasma of the ketotic patient is often hyperosmolar despite the hyponatraemia, because of the markedly raised blood-glucose.

Diabetes mellitus

Of all endocrine emergencies, those occurring in diabetic patients are the most common. Drowsiness or coma may be presenting symptoms and it is first essential to establish whether the altered state of consciousness is hypoglycaemic or hyperglycaemic in origin (Table 11.2), but the clinical differentiation is not difficult. Hypoglycaemic coma in the diabetic patient is considered subsequently with other endocrine causes of this condition.

1. Hyperglycaemia with ketoacidosis

CLINICAL FEATURES: The main features are summarized in Table 11.2. Preceding the onset of true coma there is usually epigastric discomfort, nausea and vomiting, thirst, and polyuria. Sometimes there may be severe abdominal pain which may be associated with vomiting. As the condition deteriorates there is usually some clouding of consciousness. On examination the abdomen may be rigid, mimicking an acute abdominal emergency, but urine analysis will show glycosuria and ketonuria. It is however always possible that an acute abdominal condition has precipitated the coma. Hence, it is important to assess carefully the patient's progress and if there is no improvement in the abdominal signs when the ketosis and hyperglycaemia are controlled, reassessment is essential. The classical bounding pulse of the ketotic patient is not frequently observed as the dehyration may be of such severity that the pulse is rapid and thready.

INVESTIGATIONS:

1. Whenever possible urine samples should be obtained without catheterization, to avoid possible infection. Large quantities of glucose and ketones indicate ketoacidosis, whereas marked glycosuria in the absence of ketone bodies indicate non-ketotic coma.
2. The blood-levels of glucose, urea, and electrolytes must be determined.
3. Arterial blood samples are taken to estimate pH, p_{O_2} and p_{CO_2}.
4. A haematocrit may be of some value in assessing dehyration, but usually this is determined clinically.

Table 11.2   Principal features of hyper- and hypo-glycaemic coma

	Hyperglycaemia with ketoacidosis	Hypoglycaemic
Onset	Gradual	Sudden
Precipitating factors	Infection	—
	Systemic disturbance (e.g. myocardial infarction, pancreatitis)	—
	Dietary indiscretion	Meal missed. Altered physical activity
	Insulin omitted	Insulin dose increased
	Drugs, e.g. thiazides	Oral hypoglycaemic drugs recently added to therapy β-Blocking drugs
		Onset of renal or hepatic failure
Preceding symptoms	Thirst, polyuria, weight loss, pruritus valvae, abdominal pain, tiredness, drowsiness	Hunger, cold, sweaty, giddiness and confusion
		Aggressive behaviour, palpitations, 'panic'
Signs	Dehydration, rapid deep respiration, sweet ketotic breath ('rotten apples')	Cold, sweaty, pale skin Rapid, thready pulse. Brisk reflexes and upgoing plantars
	Rapid, bounding pulse	Drowsiness, aggression, confusion, rapid onset of coma
	Depressed reflexes. Drowsiness, stupor, (gradual) coma	
Urine	Glycosuria with ketones	Usually no glycosuria

The above tests help not only to confirm the diagnosis, but also indicate the severity of the metabolic imbalance.

5. An electrocardiogram is of value to determine whether there is any cardiovascular abnormality (myocardial infarction). Subsequently it is of value to continue with a cardiac monitor, particularly if there is a past history of coronary heart disease.

6. Routine tests to identify possible infections:
   a. chest X-ray
   b. midstream urine for culture
   c. blood culture

    d. throat swabs for culture

    e. sputum examination.

Whether the patient should be nursed in an intensive care unit is debatable. In general, if there are any respiratory or cardiovascular problems, it is advisable to use such units. Despite the greater surveillance by medical and nursing staff the units are not usually utilized for the uncomplicated case of diabetic coma.

TREATMENT: It is difficult to assess whether insulin or intravenous fluid is of greater importance in the treatment of diabetic coma. It is a theoretical consideration as in practice both are employed virtually simultaneously. Fluids are discussed first in order to emphasize the importance of replenishing the deficiency in these patients.

(a) Intravenous fluid. The first litre is given as isotonic saline in 15–30 minutes. The rate of infusion is then decreased according to the degree of hydration. Usually some 6 l are given during the first 24 hours.

This simple approach assumes that there is no underlying disease such as a cardiovascular abnormality. If ischaemic heart disease is present, fluids have to be used with care and any evidence of a rise of venous pressure, or pulmonary congestion, would preclude further fluid therapy. When the blood-glucose falls below 17 mmol/l (300 mg/100 ml), dextrose–saline may be used instead of normal saline. Subsequently the patient is usually able to take fluids by mouth.

(b) Insulin. Only the short-acting insulins are used, usually insulin injection ('soluble') or neutral insulin injection (Actrapid MC); since insulin has a short half-life, frequent small doses are necessary to prevent rapid changes of plasma glucose and electrolyte concentration. The hormone is given intramuscularly or intravenously.

Intramuscular administration: Initially 15 units are given and subsequently 5–10 units/h according to the response of the patient.

Intravenous administration: Insulin at the rate of 5 units/h is infused by a constant-infusion pump. It has been suggested that an hourly intravenous bolus of 10 units of insulin into the infusing tubes may be as effective as continuous infusion.

Although intravenous administration is theoretically the method of preference, the intramuscular one is simple; furthermore it can be supplemented by an initial intravenous dose of insulin if the diabetic ketosis is severe. Both methods are effective but when the intramuscular route is used care must be taken to avoid hypoglycaemia, and to ensure adequate hydration when the intramuscular route is used.

The blood-glucose is estimated every 2–3 h and when the blood-glucose falls below 17 mmol/l (300 mg/100 ml) a sliding scale is used. The dose of insulin is determined by the urine concentration of glucose and the presence of ketones in a sample of urine tested immediately after voiding at 6-hourly intervals (Table 11.3). The insulin would thus be given once every 6 hours subcutaneously. When the 24-hour sample of urine has been collected the total insulin requirement for the next day can be calculated. This total is divided by two, with a little more than half being given in the morning and a little less than half at night, before the appropriate meal.

Table 11.3   The approximate quantities of insulin required in the immediate post-coma period, based on urinary glucose.

2% glucose*	= 24 units soluble insulin, adding 4 units for each 1+ of ketones if there is heavy ketonuria†
1% glucose	= 16 units soluble insulin; ketones are ignored
0·75% glucose	= 12 units soluble insulin; ketones are ignored
0·5% glucose	= 8 units soluble insulin; ketones are ignored

*If there is no glycosuria, 4–8 units are given before meals
†as indicated by ketodiastix

(c) Potassium. This electrolyte should be estimated at 3-hourly intervals, until the patient is conscious. Although the plasma potassium concentration may be raised when the glucose level is high, the total body potassium is often low. The blood potassium level decreases following insulin administration and this electrolyte is therefore given approximately 2 hours after the initial injection or infusion of insulin. However, the therapy is withheld if the blood potassium is raised or the cardiogram shows changes associated with hyperkalaemia. Low doses of insulin do not induce rapid shifts of potassium and therefore it is rarely necessary to infuse potassium at a rate in excess of 13 mmol chloride per hour.

(d) Sodium bicarbonate. This should not be given routinely. As a general rule bicarbonate is given only if the pH is 7·1 or less, and then a small dose (50 mmol) is administered slowly intravenously over 30 minutes; whether this should be repeated depends on the pH change. It must be emphasized that potassium is always administered at the same time unless there is an unusually severe hyperkalaemia.

(e) Treatment of precipitating factors. Infection needs prompt treatment with antibiotics. It is however important to note that leucocytosis in diabetic ketosis may be a reflection of the metabolic changes and does not necessarily indicate an infection. Nevertheless it is advisable to use a broad-spectrum antibiotic drug.

(f) General care. Regular emptying of the stomach by nasogastric tube is necessary to avoid accidental inhalation when the vomiting is severe; it also provides symptomatic relief.

2. Hyperglycaemia without ketoacidosis (hyperosmolar)

CLINICAL FEATURES: This condition is characterized by a high plasma osmolality and the resulting high viscosity may cause thrombotic complications. The blood-glucose concentration is often extremely high and values of 39 mmol/l (700 mg/100 ml) are common, but there is no significant acidosis. This condition often occurs in previously undiagnosed diabetics who may, subsequently, be stabilized by diet alone. West Indians appear to be especially prone to this disorder and the symptomatology is much the same as that of diabetic ketosis. It is interesting to note that frequently the patients refer to their previous over-indulgence in sweets and fizzy drinks. The condition is often precipitated by infection, especially of the urinary tract.

The plasma osmolality which is normally 283 ± 17 mOsmol/kg H_2O can reach a value of 350 mosmol/kg or more. If it is not possible to obtain a direct measurement of plasma osmolality, a rough estimate can be calculated by using the following formula:

†Plasma osmolality = $([Na^+]+[K^+])+[glucose]+[urea]$.

TREATMENT: This is the same as for diabetic ketosis with the following amendments.

a. Larger volumes of half-normal saline are required.
b. The total insulin requirements may be smaller.
c. Ultimately the patients often manage without insulin.
d. Anticoagulants in small dosage may be used to prevent thrombotic episodes.

3. Hyperglycaemia with lactic acidosis

This condition has a high mortality rate and in diabetic patients is often induced by phenformin, but rarely by metformin. These drugs should not be prescribed to diabetics who have renal, hepatic, or ischaemic heart disease. Indeed it is probably wise to avoid phenformin in all patients. There are many other causes of lactic acidosis, but these are not considered here.

The patient is acidotic and the diagnosis is confirmed by a lactic acid level of greater than 7 mmol/l. If this estimation is unobtainable, a presumptive diagnosis can be made by measuring the anion gap. This is obtained by adding the sodium and potassium ion concentrations and subtracting the sum of the chloride and bicarbonate concentration; this should not normally exceed 20 mmol/l.

TREATMENT: This follows the general outline presented for hyperglycaemic ketotic coma, but active correction of acid–base is more urgent and larger quantities of bicarbonate are required.

Hypoglycaemia

This may be defined as a blood-glucose concentration below 2·2 mmol/l (40 mg/100 ml), but symptoms may occur above this level in patients with diabetes mellitus. Hypoglycaemia occurs most commonly in patients with diabetes mellitus who are on insulin therapy. In patients with spontaneous hypoglycaemia, insulinoma must always be considered first. Other rare causes of this condition are Addison's disease and hypopituitarism.

CLINICAL FEATURES: It is important to recall that patients with autonomic neuropathy may lapse into coma without symptoms, and such signs as sweating may be absent. In this section certain specialized clinical aspects are emphasized. The patients may show interesting changes in personality prior to the onset of coma. There may be impairment of the so-called 'higher centres' with the appearance of a 'drunk-like state' (e.g. slurring of speech, aggressiveness, impairment of routine acts, somnolence). More marked personality defects may occur in patients who have had many hypoglycaemic attacks previously; sometimes dementia or psychosis may occur.

† SI units must be used.

There may be neurological changes, for example monoplegia associated with an extensor plantar response (Babinski sign). Diabetic patients who have the added complications of renal and/or hepatic disease are prone to hypoglycaemia. In children, infants, and particularly premature infants, convulsions may be the presenting feature.

INVESTIGATIONS: Classically the blood-glucose concentration is below 2·2 mmol/l (40 mg/100 ml) and a blood sample should be taken immediately, prior to therapy. Use of a Dextrostix provides a quick and valuable test for hypoglycaemia, but it is essential that the sticks are fresh.

TREATMENT: Without delay 10–20 ml of a 50% dextrose solution is given; recovery is usually immediate. However, if the coma has been of many hours' duration it may persist despite the glucose therapy. It is probably a wise procedure to treat all unconscious patients in whom the diagnosis is uncertain in this manner, since the administration of glucose can do no harm. Within 30 minutes the results of the plasma glucose level are available. If the diagnosis is confirmed and the patient is still unconscious or confused, further intravenous glucose should be given and glucagon 1 μg may be given intramuscularly. If the patient recovers consciousness 20 g oral glucose is given.

Occasionally hypoglycaemia can be refractory and the long-acting sulphonylurea drugs (chlorpropamide and glibenclamide) may be responsible. In these circumstances it is necessary to infuse the glucose intravenously until the patient is conscious. It must be emphasized that the treatment of hypoglycaemia is an emergency because neurological damage is related to the period of unconsciousness.

Subsequent treatment depends on the aetiology of the hypoglycaemia. In the case of the diabetic patient, adjustment of the dose of insulin or the diet may be necessary; if the patient has omitted a meal the importance of following the diabetic regimen must be emphasized. The appropriate treatment for the other conditions is considered in the relevant chapters.

Myxoedema coma

This rare condition usually occurs in the elderly when the environmental temperature is low.

CLINICAL FEATURES: Specific clinical features which characterize this disease are usually present (see Chapter 6). However, hypothermia of the elderly may often resemble myxoedema coma and differentiation of the two conditions is difficult.

Hypothermia is present in 50 per cent of patients with myxoedema coma and is arbitrarily defined as a core temperature (rectal temperature) below 35 °C. If the temperature is not low, there is probably an underlying infection which may easily escape recognition. It must be emphasized that in order to detect the hypothermia it is essential to use a low-reading thermometer which has been adequately shaken.

Apart from the coma, other important features of this condition can be summarized as follows: hypoventilation associated with carbon dioxide retention, hypotension, and bradycardia, preceded sometimes by psychotic changes.

INVESTIGATIONS:

1. The plasma levels of T_4 and TSH are determined. A very low T_4 and high TSH establish the diagnosis. Unfortunately, these results may not be available for two to three days. As the treatment is urgent the diagnosis has to be made on clinical grounds

2. It is of value to determine the arterial po_2 and pco_2, as frequently the patient is not distressed even when these are considerably disturbed.

3. Whether blood electrolytes should be estimated if the therapy includes cortisol is debatable, but this investigation may result in a more comprehensive knowledge of the disease. For example, the cause of the occasionally observed hyponatraemia in this condition is not yet fully understood.

TREATMENT:

a. A small dose of T_3 (20 μg) is given intravenously at 12-h intervals. Once consciousness has returned the patient receives sufficient oral T_4 to restore the euthyroid state.

b. Hydrocortisone hemisuccinate (100 mg) is given intravenously every 12 hours. This therapy is advocated because it is sometimes difficult to distinguish between the coma due to myxoedema and that due to hypopituitarism. In addition, the response to stress in myxoedema may be impaired.

c. As respiration is often depressed, it is essential that the airway be maintained and if necessary artificial ventilation is given.

d. Gradual rewarming is achieved by heating the air surrounding the patient, with an electric blanket over a cradle, at a rate of about $0 \cdot 5 \, °C/h$.

e. Fluids are restricted as hyponatraemia is often present.

f. General care:
   i. respiratory depressants should be avoided and great care exercised with all drugs that are administered, as metabolism is much slower.
   ii. a cardiac monitor is used for the detection of cardiac arrhythmias, and the low voltage of the complexes can be observed.

Hypopituitary coma

This may present in patients with a past history of postpartum haemorrhage followed by failure to lactate and amenorrhoea (Sheehans' syndrome). It may be precipitated by a cold environment in patients with mild hypopituitarism.

CLINICAL FEATURES: These patients may present in an exactly similar manner to those with myxoedema coma or with acute adrenal cortical failure. However, in addition there is usually evidence of gonadal insufficiency, for example loss of pubic and axillary hair, and pale skin. Table 11.4 summarizes these changes. While hypothermia is frequently observed, hypoglycaemia of sufficient severity to induce symptoms is not common.

INVESTIGATIONS: Plasma levels of cortisol, T_4, and all trophic hormones, are estimated. The typical changes are a low T_4 and a low TSH.

Table 11.4   Effects of trophic hormone deficiency

Gonadotrophins	TSH	ACTH	General changes
Loss of pubic and axillary hair	Loss of energy; cold-intolerance	Pale skin	Anaemia, apathy, and depression
Amenorrhoea	Dry brittle hair; baldness	Hypoglycaemia	
Testicular atrophy. Loss of libido. Fine facial hair	Voice normal (cf. myxoedema)	Poor response to stress	

TREATMENT:

a. If hypoglycaemia is present, the treatment is as previously described.

b. Hydrocortisone hemisuccinate (100 mg) is given intravenously (and subsequently intramuscularly) as soon as possible. This is then replaced by oral therapy.

c. It may be necessary to administer thyroid hormones as described for myxoedema.

Addisonian crisis

This condition usually occurs in a patient with known adrenal insufficiency who develops a superimposed infection or is exposed to some stress such as a surgical procedure without adequate supplementation of exogenous hormone. The crisis is often precipitated by further shrinkage of extracellular volume following diarrhoea and vomiting. Sometimes the patient may present in hypoglycaemic coma. The disease may present for the first time.

CLINICAL FEATURES: There is severe prostration, weakness, and hypotension in addition to the diarrhoea and vomiting. These patients may or may not have stigmata of chronic adrenal insufficiency (see Table 11.5) and may have signs of the underlying aetiology. A rare but interesting example of acute adrenal failure occurs in meningococcal septicaemia (Waterhouse–Friderichsen syndrome) which is associated with a purpuric rash.

INVESTIGATIONS:

1. Plasma levels of electrolytes and urea are estimated; typical changes are raised plasma urea, hyperkalaemia, and hyponatraemia.

2. The plasma cortisol and ACTH concentrations are determined.

Unfortunately the hormone concentration estimations may not be available for several days and, since treatment is urgent, the diagnosis is usually based on clinical grounds and the characteristic electrolyte changes.

TREATMENT:

a. One litre of normal saline is given intravenously in the first hour and

Table 11.5   Changes observed in adrenal cortical deficiency

Cortisol deficiency	Aldosterone deficiency	Other changes
Hypotension	Excess sodium excretion; hyponatraemia	Nausea and vomiting
Extreme weakness		Anorexia and weight loss
Hypoglycaemia	Excess potassium retention; hyperkalaemia	Diarrhoea
Low glomerular filtration rate and uraemia		
Increased ACTH secretion; pigmentation		

subsequently the rate is decreased; dextrose saline is now used. The total quantity and the rate of infusion are determined by the state of dehydration and the blood-pressure. About 4 l are required during the first 24 hours.

b. Hydrocortisone hemisuccinate (100 mg) is given intravenously and repeated every 8 h, as necessary. It is advantageous to establish an intravenous infusion before administering the hydrocortisone since intravenous injection may be extremely difficult. As soon as the condition improves the patient is given oral replacement therapy; most patients are stabilized with 30 mg of cortisol a day (20 mg in the morning and 10 mg at night).

c. Antibiotic therapy is administered if an infection is the precipitating or causal factor.

Hypocalcaemia

This condition may present as coma if it is associated with hyperventilation, generalized convulsion, or tetany. It must be emphasized that tetany is more frequently observed in patients with alkalosis without hypocalcaemia (the commonest cause being overbreathing in patients with hysteria). Other causes of tetany may be hypokalaemia or hypomagnesaemia.

CLINICAL FEATURES: There may be a history of cramps and parasthesiae and the clinical signs of tetany followed by convulsions may have preceded this coma. The coma is of short duration, possibly being terminated by a fall in blood pH, as carbon dioxide accumulates during the period of apnoea. The convulsions may present in a fashion which is indistinguishable from grand mal or petit mal. Furthermore patients with hypocalcaemia may have papilloedema in which case the differential diagnosis is difficult. In infants or children hypocalcaemia may present as fits often heralded by laryngeal stridor (crowing inspiration).

INVESTIGATIONS:

1. The blood calcium level is determined and the ionized calcium is usually below 1·2 mmol/l (5mg/100 ml), if this measurement is available.
2. The blood pH is of value to exclude alkalaemia.
3. The plasma potassium and magnesium levels are estimated.

TREATMENT: This depends on the coma, but routinely 10–30 ml of 10% calcium gluconate in 500–1500 ml of isotonic saline is administered intravenously.

Hypercalcaemia

Metastatic carcinoma is the commonest cause of hypercalcaemia and although it rarely presents as an emergency it is worthy of note as there are some interesting features.

CLINICAL FEATURES: Patients with hypercalcaemia may present in coma. There is often a history of malaise, headaches, abdominal pain, constipation, anorexia, and vomiting. The coma is preceded by drowsiness which slowly deepens. There is hypotension associated with dehydration.

INVESTIGATIONS:

1. The plasma calcium concentration is determined and this is usually above 4·2 mmol/l (17 mg/100 ml); frequently there is hypokalaemia. The blood calcium estimation should be repeated during treatment. If this investigation is not freely available, cardiograms may be used by measuring the 'corrected' QT period (QT_c). Fig 11.1 illustrates how this is obtained. It is claimed that the blood calcium is inversely proportional to the QT_c interval.
2. Renal function is assessed by estimating plasma urea, creatinine, and phosphate concentrations.

TREATMENT:

a. If the patient is on therapy which would induce a positive calcium balance, this should be stopped.
b. Intravenous saline infusion frequently corrects the dehydration and markedly improves the condition.

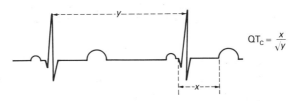

$$QT_c = \frac{x}{\sqrt{y}}$$

Fig.11.1   Measurement of the corrected QT period (QT_c) of a cardiogram.

c. Intravenous infusion of frusemide together with isotonic saline increases calcium excretion. If the three treatments listed above are unsuccessful, other measures may be used.

d. Fifteen mmol of phosphate infused intravenously over 6–8 hours.

e. Steroids (60–80 mg initially) are especially helpful if the hypercalcaemia is due to sarcoidosis or vitamin D intoxication and it may be beneficial in malignant conditions. There is a long latent period of 5–7 days before this therapy lowers the plasma calcium concentration.

f. Haemodialysis may be of value when other measures fail. It is also used if renal failure is present.

g. Calcitonin (5–25 μg/kg) may be of therapeutic value.

h. Methramycin should be used only as a last resort, as it is a toxic substance which damages the liver and kidneys and impairs platelet function. In addition there may be severe local reactions.

Thyroid crisis

This may occur in thyrotoxic patients 24–48 hours after thyroidectomy and in untreated thyrotoxic patients who have an intercurrent infection. Some common precipitating factors are hyperglycaemic ketotic coma, toxaemia of pregnancy, and parturition.

CLINICAL FEATURES: There is a marked pyrexia and exacerbation of the features of thyrotoxicosis (see Chapter 6). Dehydration, particularly if the environmental temperature is high, may be marked. Nausea, vomiting, and abdominal pain may be early symptoms. The pulse rate may be very rapid and atrial fibrillation can occur with cardiac failure. In addition, apathy can be severe and the patient may progress to stupor or even coma. Thyroid crisis requires urgent treatment.

INVESTIGATIONS: There are no routine tests and diagnosis is based on the clinical picture.

TREATMENT:

a. Antithyroid drugs given orally or by intramuscular injection.

b. Iodides by mouth, 10 mg every 6 hours.

c. A β-blocker such as propranolol (10–40 mg 6-hourly) to reduce sympathetic activity; this therapy should be used in conjunction with a cardiac monitor.

d. A litre of dextrose–saline is given intravenously in 1–2 hours; subsequently the quantity depends on the severity of the dehydration.

e. Hydrocortisone (100–300 mg daily) is a valuable supportive measure.

f. Tepid sponging if there is hyperpyrexia.

g. Sedation using any of the standard preparations.

Hypertensive crisis in phaeochromocytoma

This tumour may present as an acute emergency and is considered only briefly in this section. There may be severe paroxysmal or sustained hypertension which may progress to a cardiovascular accident or cardiac arrhythmias; occasionally diarrhoea may precipitate severe dehydration (see p. 41). The patient may be extremely distressed by the unpleasant sensation of 'panic'.

INVESTIGATIONS: In an acute emergency usually only the phentolamine test is used (see Chapter 3).

TREATMENT: It is essential to reduce blood-pressure and increase plasma volume with α-blockers such as phenoxybenzamine which may be given as 1 mg/kg body weight in an intravenous infusion of 5 per cent glucose over a period of 2 hours. Subsequently β-blockers such as propranalol can then be used to control the tachycardia.

12 Tests of endocrine function

In this chapter a brief consideration of the radioimmunoassay is followed by specific tests of endocrine function. Notes on the handling and transport to assay laboratories of biological fluids, together with other relevant information, are readily available in the handbook provided by the Supra-Regional Assay Service (SRAS) which can be found in any Regional assay laboratory.

Since it is impossible to consider all endocrine function tests in a book of this size we have limited the number of conditions discussed to those which present most commonly. The inclusion of actual examples which show characteristic changes in hormone levels for the conditions discussed will, we hope, prove to be useful to the reader.

The radioimmunoassay

The determination of hormonal concentrations in biological fluids has advanced knowledge not only of the physiology of endocrine glands, but also of disorders in their function. Of the various methods used to assay the concentration of hormones in body fluids, the radioimmunoassay is generally the most successful. Unfortunately, because of the use and success of this technique diagnosis is sometimes made only on the basis of the radioimmunoassay results and all clinical acumen is abandoned; this reveals a basic defect in the understanding of the assay because of an insufficient awareness of its limitations. It is therefore important to realize that the measurement of a hormone concentration is not itself directly indicative of the presence (or absence) of a disease, but provides an extremely useful guideline in confirming or excluding that disease.

Principles of the technique

The radioimmunoassay depends on the principle that a hormone can act like an antigen in certain circumstances, so that a specific antibody for that hormone can be developed. It may be that the hormone itself is non-antigenic (e.g. a steroid), in which case it is necessary to form a complex between the hormone and, for example, albumin; the complex can then act as a suitable antigen. A standard preparation of the purified hormone can be labelled with a radioisotope and a known amount added to a known quantity of antibody. To this mixture may now be added the unlabelled test hormone. The degree of binding of the antibody with the labelled hormone is a measure of the concentration of the unlabelled hormone present (see Fig. 12.1).

By measuring the radioactivity in the bound antibody-labelled hormone

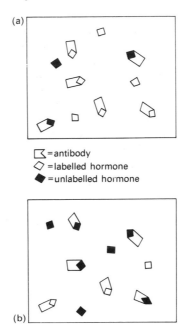

Fig.12.1 The binding of antibody to labelled and unlabelled hormone antigen: (a) when excess labelled (standard) hormone is present; and (b) when excess unlabelled (test) hormone is present.

fraction, an estimate of the concentration of the unlabelled (test) hormone can then be obtained. In order to obtain this estimate, a standard curve for the hormone being investigated is necessary. To plot this curve a series of responses is obtained by adding various known concentrations of unlabelled standard hormone to mixtures containing known quantities of labelled standard hormone and the specific antibody (see Fig. 12.2). Any one standard curve allows for the assay of the hormone within a range which may extend over a sixfold increase in concentration. By altering the quantity of antibody in the mixture of labelled and unlabelled hormone, the range of sensitivities can be varied. Thus one can provide a suitable series of standard curves, each curve for a particular range. For example, it can be seen from the curve in Fig. 12.2 that for a change in concentration of unlabelled hormone from 6mU to 1 mU, the percentage of antibody bound to labelled hormone falls from 70 to 20 per cent. If 0·1 ml of the sample containing unlabelled hormone is assayed, it may be seen from the curve that the percentage of bound labelled antibody is 50 per cent. This will give a value of 2·3 mU of the unlabelled hormone and hence a concentration of 23 mU/ml. In this way the graph can be used to obtain the concentration of hormone in serum if it falls within the range of this curve. In order to achieve a satisfactory radioimmunoassay for a particular hormone there are the following prerequisites:

1. A purified hormone preparation for use as the standard; this may not always be obtainable. The term 'pure' is often applied even when it is known that some impurity may be present, so that in practice a hormone preparation with the highest purity available is used as standard.

2. A specific antibody with sufficient affinity for the hormone. Some hormones may not themselves be antigens, in which case strategies such as reacting the hormone with some other molecule, e.g. a protein, have to be used in order to confer antigenic properties on that molecule.

3. A satisfactory technique for separating the bound hormone–antibody fraction from the free component.

The principle of the radioimmunoassay also applies to competitive protein-binding assays in which labelled and unlabelled hormone fractions compete for protein (carrier) molecules which act as 'antibodies'. The principal hormones for which this competitive protein-binding is used as an assay technique are cortisol and thyroxine. For example, labelled (standard) cortisol and unlabelled (test) cortisol will both compete for transcortin molecules. Separation of free from bound components (e.g. with charcoal), followed by radioimmunoassay of the bound fraction will give an estimate of the relative

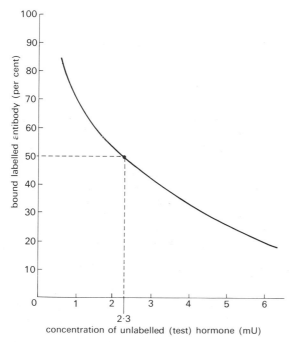

Fig.12.2 Standard curve covering a range of 1–6 mU for the concentration of unlabelled (test) hormone related to the percentage of antibody bound to labelled (standard) hormone.

proportions of labelled to unlabelled hormone. The degree of binding is then a measure of the concentration of the test hormone as discussed previously.

Limitations of the technique

The radioimmunoassay is a technique which has generally improved the ease of measuring the concentrations of many biological substances, but unfortunately there are various technical problems which nevertheless can limit its present application. For instance the problem of delineating the absolute specificity of the antibody in many instances remains unresolved. Biological activity (as determined by a bioassay) for a particular hormone may not be identical to the activity of that hormone as measured using a radioimmunoassay for many reasons (e.g. poor antibody specificity, or to an impure standard hormone preparation, etc.). One well-documented example is the radioimmunoassay for insulin, which measures not only the concentration of insulin, but also of proinsulin, also present in the blood. This precursor molecule has only about 10 per cent of the biological activity of insulin, but both molecules will be labelled and both react with the antibody so that the estimation of insulin concentration will be misleadingly high in the radioimmunoassay.

Specific limitations

1. Protein and peptide hormones

a. Sample stability: many of the protein and peptide hormones have relatively long half-lives and are therefore fairly stable. For these hormones (e.g. thyrotrophin, luteinizing hormone, and follicle-stimulating hormone) no special precautions are needed. For those hormones which have short half-lives (e.g. corticotrophin, parathormone, and insulin), plasma samples should be frozen within 10 minutes of venepuncture.

b. Precision: most radioimmunoassays are accurate within 10–20 per cent (coefficient of variation). If for example, a value of 100 U/ml was obtained for a particular hormone concentration and the coefficient of variation was 10 per cent for that radioimmunoassay, then it could be said that the actual value was somewhere between 90 and 110 U/ml.

c. Sensitivity: the radioimmunoassay cannot measure concentrations at the lower end of the normal range or sub-normal levels for some hormones (e.g. corticotrophin, thyrotrophin, and parathormone). For example, the diagnosis of thyrotoxicosis cannot, therefore, be confirmed by measurement of thyrotrophin levels.

d. Specificity: an important point to note is that for some radioimmunoassays, the antibody recognizes only a small part of the antigenic molecule and therefore cross-reactivity between similar polypeptides or fragments of similar molecules can occur (e.g. between insulin and proinsulin molecules).

2. Steroids and other hormones transported bound to globulins

Most steroids (e.g. cortisol and testosterone) and certain other hormones (e.g.

the thyroid hormones T_3 and T_4) are normally transported in the blood bound to specific plasma globulins (e.g. transcortin for cortisol, sex-hormone binding globulin SHBG for testosterone, and thyroxine-binding globulin TBG). Most assays measure total hormone activity (bound and free fractions) and therefore when the binding globulin concentration is altered total hormone activity may be misleading, since it is the free hormone component which is physiologically active and this may be within the normal range. For example, patients on the contraceptive pill may have a raised TBG level (in which case the total T_4 concentration will be raised) but the·free hormone level will be normal and the patient euthyroid. Another example would be a male patient with thyrotoxicosis complaining of impotence. The total testosterone level may actually be found to be raised due to T_4 stimulating hepatic SHBG synthesis; free testosterone would nevertheless be reduced.

a. Sample stability: steroids (and thyroid hormones) are relatively stable in blood and therefore no special precautions are required provided that samples are centrifuged at 4 °C within 24 hours.

b. Precision: the coefficient of variation is usually less than 10 per cent.

c. Sensitivity: present methodology is adequate for the detection of subnormal levels of hormone by radioimmunoassay.

d. Specificity: the radioimmunoassays are usually relatively specific but occasionally can be improved by purification of samples by chromatography prior to the assay.

Note: Not all hormone estimations are routinely made using radioimmunoassays. Cortisol, for example, is still estimated by the fluorimetric technique in the majority of laboratories. The main problem associated with this assay is that aldactone gives spurious results. Cortisol levels measured using this technique in patients with hypertension being treated with this drug are therefore erroneous. However, radioimmunoassay can always be used to confirm diagnosis in such a situation. Another assay technique, gas chromatography, is increasingly being replaced by the radioimmunoassay.

SPECIFIC TESTS OF ENDOCRINE FUNCTION

Neurohypophysial function

Diabetes insipidus

Plasma osmolality is usually raised from the normal value of 280 ± 6 (S.D) to 295 ± 15 (S.D) mosm/kg. Urine is hypo-osmolar (less than 300 mosm/kg H_2O and sometimes as low as 50 mosm/kg H_2O). The plasma and urine osmolalities are generally estimated following dehydration and vasopressin tests.

Syndrome of Inappropriate ADH (SIADH)

Measured plasma sodium concentrations are usually below normal (hyponatraemia) and are often lower than 120 mmol/l. Plasma potassium and protein concentrations are usually decreased (haemodilution). Urinary (or plasma) vasopressin levels can be estimated by radioimmunoassay or by bioassay, and if raised this confirms the diagnosis. It is important to note that hyponatraemia is not always associated with raised vasopressin concentrations. Normal values for vasopressin levels are:

plasma vasopressin concentration: 1–2 μU/ml

urine vasopressin excretion (resting subjects):   10 mU/24 h

urine vasopressin excretion (normal activity):   usually 10–40 mU/24 h.

(The urinary vasopressin concentration is dependent upon the level of activity of the subject or patient.)

Adenohypophysial function

COMBINED PITUITARY FUNCTION TEST: The recommended procedure for determining adenohypophysial function is called the combined pituitary function test. It includes the simultaneous administration of thyrotrophin-releasing hormone (TRH), LH releasing hormone (LHRH), and insulin-induced hypoglycaemia. The insulin-induced hypoglycaemia is used for investigating somatotrophin, prolactin, and corticotrophin secretion. The combined pituitary function test should not be carried out on patients over 60 years old, or on patients with cardiovascular problems or a history of fits.

Procedure: The patient is fasted overnight but allowed free access to water. The test is done between 0800 and 1000 h, before breakfast. It is recommended that the patient should be lying down comfortably. An indwelling venous catheter such as a G19 Butterfly with a three-way tap is inserted. The catheter can be kept patent with saline which can be heparinized. After an initial rest period of half an hour, a basal blood sample is taken. Soluble insulin is then administered in a recommended dose of 0·15 U/kg body weight. In patients already suspected of hypopituitarism the dose can be reduced to 0·1 U/kg while for patients with acromegaly it can be increased to 0·3 U/kg. The two hormones LHRH and TRH are given simultaneously as an intravenous bolus in doses of 100 μg and 200 μg respectively. A blood-sample is then taken every 15 minutes for the first hour and every 30 minutes for the second hour.

Hypoglycaemia usually occurs 35–50 minutes after injection, the symptoms and signs being mainly sweating, headaches, raised blood-pressure and increased heart-rate. The blood-glucose concentration usually decreases to below 2·2 mmol/l. The hypoglycaemia lasts for 15–20 minutes. At the end of the test, the patient, who generally feels very hungry, should get a full breakfast.

If the hypoglycaemia has not occurred within 1 hour the same dose of insulin can be repeated. Some patients may suffer severe hypoglycaemic symptoms and in these circumstances it is advisable to give 50 ml of 50% dextrose solution, which should be readily available at the bedside. It is important to note that once hypoglycaemia has occurred, the appropriate blood samples should still be taken despite the possible necessity of infusing the glucose solution.

The various blood-samples are then analysed and the concentrations of glucose and various hormones are estimated. In Table 12.1, values obtained for a normal person given the combined pituitary function test are given as an example.

Results: In order to interpret the results it is necessary to know the normal basal values for the concentrations of the various substances estimated. These are:

Glucose concentration (fasting)	3·0–5·0 mmol/l
T₄	60 160 nmol/l
T₃	1·4–3·0 nmol/l
Thyrotrophin (TSH)	up to 5 mU/l
Prolactin (PRL)	up to 800 mU/l
LH (female, follicular phase)	2·5–15·0 U/l
FSH (female, follicular phase)	1–10 U/l
Somatotrophin (HGH in fasting, non-stressed patient)	less than 0·5 mU/l
Cortisol (0900 h)	250–700 nmol/l

In the example of a normal patient (Table 12.1) hypoglycaemia occurred within 15 minutes, the blood glucose level being below 2·2 mmol/l. The patient showed various symptoms of hypoglycaemia 30 minutes after the intravenous injection, lasting for approximately 30 minutes. In response to the hypoglycaemia there was:

(a) an increase in cortisol concentration of more than 250 nmol/l from the basal value at 60–90 minutes post-injection;

(b) a rise in the somatotrophin (HGH) level to above 40 mU/l at 60–90 minutes post-injection;

(c) an increase in prolactin in response to the hypoglycaemia masked by the response to TRH.

Table 12.1. Example of normal combined pituitary function test†

Time	Glucose	T₄	T₃	TSH	PRL	Cortisol	LH	FSH	HGH
(min)	(mmol/)	(nmol/l)		(mU/l)	(mU/l)	(nmol/l)	(U/l)	(U/l)	(mU/l)
0	4·3	88	2·0	<1·5	200	350	1·6	2·6	<0·5
10 U soluble insulin; 200 µg TRH; 100 µg LHRH given as i.v. bolus at 0 time									
15	1·3	—	—	3·9	1080	355	10·9	6·0	<0·5
30	1·4	—	—	3·5	1800	390	16·7	10·2	13
45	1·7	—	—	2·5	2000	480	11·4	8·3	60
60	2·1	—	—	2·5	1800	640	9·7	8·0	84
90	2·5	—	—	—	1200	640	—	—	54
120	3·0	—	—	—	702	460	—	—	24

† Female (in follicular phase): weight = 70 kg.

In response to the 200 μg TRH:

(a) an increase in thyrotrophin (TSH) concentration up to 3–15 mU/l should occur some 20 minutes after injection. The value observed at 15 minutes (3·9 mU/l) was within this range;

(b) the normal increase in prolactin (PRL) level in response to TRH has not yet been defined, but in 12 normal subjects investigated at Charing Cross Hospital the mean prolactin level 20 minutes after injection was 1800 mU/l.

In response to 100 μg LHRH, there was:

(a) an increase in LH levels to within an expected range of 15–42 U/l approximately 20 minutes after injection (16·7 U/l at 30 minutes);

(b) an increase in FSH levels; the expected range for such an increase in response to the injection of LHRH has not yet been determined.

By contrast, Table 12.2 gives the values found in a patient with a chromophobe adenoma before hypophysectomy.

Table 12.2   Example of pituitary function test on a patient with a chromophobe adenoma before hypophysectomy

Time	Glucose	T₄	T₃	TSH	PRL	Cortisol	LH	FSH	HGH
(min)	(mmol/l)	(nmol/l)		(mU/l)	(mU/l)	(nmol/l)	(U/l)	(U/l)	(mU/l)
0	*4·7*	*73*	*2·1*	*<2*	*1480*	*405*	*5·5*	*5·9*	*<0·5*
15	2·4	—	—	5	2000	335	14·9	9·7	<0·5
30	1·7	—	—	5	1940	235	21·2	9·6	<0·5
45	1·6	—	—	4	1760	235	21·7	10·7	<0·5
60	3·0	—	—	4	1700	600	19·7	9·2	1·0
90	3·5	—	—	—	1440	550	—	—	0·9
120	3·9	—	—	—	1280	350	—	—	<0·5

In this example the interpretation of results is:

(a) in the basal blood sample (0 time) the only abnormality detected is the high prolactin level;

(b) the insulin hypoglycaemia induced a normal cortisol response but there was no somatotrophin (HGH) response;

(c) the TRH induced a normal thyrotrophin (TSH) response, and prolactin increased;

(d) LHRH: both LH and FSH responses were normal.

In a series of 10 patients with pituitary tumours, the pituitary function test gave certain consistent findings. These were: (i) a high prolactin level, which in some patients rose in response to TRH; (ii) a lack of response by somato-trophin to hypoglycaemia; (iii) some patients showed a decreased response by LH and FSH to LHRH; (iv) normal thyrotrophin responses to TRH in all

Table 12.3 Example of pituitary function test carried out on a patient with a chromophobe adenoma after hypophysectomy

Time	Glucose	T_4	T_3	TSH	PRL	Cortisol	LH	FSH	HGH
(min)	(mmol/l)	(nmol/l)		(mU/l)	(mU/l)	(nmol/l)	(U/l)	(U/l)	(mU/l)
0	*3·3*	*81*	*2·4*	*3*	*1000*	*90*	*3·7*	*6·2*	*<0·5*
15	2·0	—	—	6	1160	150	6·4	5·5	<0·5
30	1·0	—	—	6	1500	80	10·9	9·1	<0·5
45	1·8	—	—	4	1400	190	13·7	8·0	0·7
60	1·9	—	—	4	1160	290	11·5	9·5	1·0
90	2·0	—	—		1160	280			1·0
120	3·1	—	—		1040	170			0·8

patients. The cortisol response to hypoglycaemia was normal in 9 out of the 10 patients. Table 12.3 shows the results of the combined pituitary function test in the same patient (see Table 12.2) with a chromophobe adenoma, after hypophysectomy.

This patient did not require long-term steroid or thyroid hormone replacement therapy.

Hypersecretion of somatotrophin

To test for acromegaly, a glucose tolerance test (GTT) is carried out. The patient is fasted overnight. Between 0800 and 1000 h a basal blood sample is taken and 50 g of glucose given orally. Blood samples are then taken every 30 minutes for 2 hours. Glucose and somatotrophin concentrations are estimated in each sample. A normal subject has a normal GTT curve and somatotrophin is depressed to less than 2 mU/l after the glucose administration.

An example of the type of response one can find in a patient with acromegaly is given in Table 12.4. In this patient there is a paradoxical rise in the somatotrophin concentration, an observation found in only a small proportion of acromegalics. The diagnosis of acromegaly is confirmed by the finding that the

Table 12.4 Example of the results of a glucose tolerance test in a patient with acromegaly

Time (min)	Glucose (mmol/l)	HGH (mU/l)
0	*7·4*	*15·3*
50 g glucose given orally at 0 time		
30	14·2	19·5
60	14·9	20·0
90	15·1	52·0
120	12·9	24·0

somatotrophin is not suppressed to a concentration less than 2 mU/l after oral glucose.

Hyposecretion of somatotrophin

Patients with complete absence of somatotrophin fail to show a rise in the somatotrophin level after insulin-induced hypoglycaemia. A partial deficiency will result in a slight increase in the concentration of somatotrophin but the value reached will be less than 40 mU/l.

To test for deficiency of HGH in young children the exercise test can be applied. For this test the child undergoes severe exercise (e.g. with the use of a cycle ergometer). The plasma somatotrophin level is investigated 5 and 20 minutes after the exercise period. If the hormone level has not reached 20 mU/l, the insulin-hypoglycaemia test is then carried out to confirm the diagnosis.

Adrenal medulla function

Hypersecretion of catecholamines

To diagnose a patient with phaeochromocytoma, the urinary vanillyl mandelic acid (VMA) concentration is measured in five consecutive 24-hour periods. If the concentration is high (for normal levels see Reference Table, p. 212) the diagnosis is confirmed. If the VMA concentration is normal or low and yet the belief that a phaeochromocytoma is still strong, the plasma and urinary concentrations of the catecholamines are estimated.

Adrenal cortex function

Hypersecretion of cortisol (Cushing's syndrome)

To diagnose this condition a screening test is recommended. This consists of morning and evening estimations of the plasma cortisol level. At midnight the patient is then given 1 mg of dexamethasone orally, and another plasma cortisol level estimation is carried out the following morning. After the blood-sample has been taken, 250 μg of synacthen is administered by either intra-muscular or intravenous injection; another blood-sample is taken for plasma cortisol estimation 30 minutes later. Initial morning and evening cortisol values will indicate the presence (or absence) of a diurnal variation. Normally, the evening level is lower than the morning value.

The synacthen test indicates the responsiveness of the adrenals to corticotrophin; the dexamethasone test indicates whether hypophysial corticotrophin can still be inhibited. It is important to note that depressive patients, some obese patients, or patients who are very stressed (e.g. hospitalized) may all show loss of diurnal variation and increased cortisol production as indicated by urinary free cortisol concentrations. The dexamethasone suppression test is therefore a necessary part of the screening procedure. Table 12.5 gives values for the plasma cortisol levels to be expected following the screening procedure for Cushing's syndrome in a normal control patient and in a patient with the condition.

Table 12.5 **Examples of results of Cushing's syndrome screening test: cortisol levels in nmol/l**

	Cushing's syndrome patient	Normal range
DAY 1		
a.m.	480	560
p.m.	500	200
Midnight: 1 mg dexamethasone given		
DAY 2		
a.m.	570	175
250 µg synacthen given		
30 minutes post-synacthen	750	560

Note: Λ positive screening test for Cushing's syndrome should be confirmed by X-ray investigations of the skull and abdomen and an intravenous pyelogram.

Differental diagnosis

Once Cushing's syndrome has been established in a patient, a differential diagnosis is necessary to determine whether the cause is a pituitary adenoma, an adrenal adenoma or carcinoma, or the ectopic production of corticotrophin (usually from an oat-cell carcinoma of the lung). An example of the cortisol levels estimated in a patient with a corticotrophin (ACTH)-producing pituitary tumour is given in Table 12.6.

Table 12.6 **An example of cortisol levels (nmol/l) levels in a patient with a pituitary tumour producing corticotrophin**

	Levels in patient	Normal range
DAY 1		
Morning	550	250–750
Midnight	660	up to 220
Midnight: 1 mg dexamethasone given		
DAY 2		
a.m. post-dexamethasone	496	<200
250 mg synacthen given (intramuscularly)		
30 minutes post-synacthen	1320	
24-hour urine analysis		
17-oxogenic steroids	26 µmol	
17-oxosteroids	69 µmol	
Free cortisol	1400 nmol	

An exaggerated synacthen test may be used, but the more common differentiation tests are the prolonged dexamethasone suppression test and the metyrapone test.

PROLONGED DEXAMETHASONE SUPPRESSION TEST: In this test 2 mg dexamethasone are given every 6 hours. In the normal subject the serum corticosteroid concentration is drastically decreased and by the third day is usually less than 50 per cent of a control value. In a patient with adrenal hyperplasia (due to a hypophysial tumour) the serum cortisol level will have decreased but is usually only reduced by some 20–30 per cent of basal values. Patients with adrenal tumours show no suppression of serum cortisol levels by this test. It is important to remember that certain drugs, particularly aldactone, interfere with serum corticosteroid estimations, and should not be given for several days before the test.

The urinary 24-hour excretion of 17-oxogenic steroids and 17-oxosteroids may be used as estimates of adrenocortical function instead of, or in addition to, free cortisol levels.

Normal 24-hour values are:

Urinary free cortisol	up to 275 nmol
17-oxosteroids	(male) 15–85 μmol; (female) 15–70 μmol
17-oxogenic steroids	(male) 15–70 μmol; (female) 15–60 μmol

METYRAPONE TEST: This drug blocks 11-hydroxylase activity and therefore the plasma cortisol concentration decreases; precursor metabolite concentrations (e.g. 17-oxosteroids and 17-oxogenic steroids) increase, however. In addition, hypophysial corticotrophin secretion should increase as the negative feedback by cortisol is reduced. If the cause of Cushing's syndrome is a pituitary tumour, then plasma corticotrophin levels and the urinary excretion of 17-oxo- and oxogenic steroids increase. If the syndrome is caused by an adrenal adenoma or carcinoma there is no rise in the excretion of these substances.

Procedure: Metyrapone (750 mg) is given orally every 4 hours for 24 hours in a patient weighing 70 kg or more. Urines should be collected for the two 24-hour periods before the drug is given, the test 24 hours and the following 24 hours. Plasmas should be taken immediately before the test and every hour for 4 hours after the first dose of drug.

Ectopic corticotrophin secretion

In patients in which excess corticotrophin secretion is produced ectopically, the hormone level is extremely high. Diagnosis is usually made by estimating corticotrophin concentrations, and by the presence of a hypokalaemic alkalosis.

Hypersecretion of aldosterone (Conn's syndrome)

The patient with Conn's syndrome has hypertension. The electrolyte pattern found is: high plasma sodium, low potassium, and high bicarbonate concentrations (hypokalaemic alkalosis). The patient will have high plasma and urine aldosterone levels on a diet with normal sodium and potassium (Na^+: 100–200 mmol/24 h; K^+: 50–80 mmol/24 h). Plasma renin activity should be low. A high salt diet does not suppress the plasma and urine aldosterone concentrations.

Hyposecretion of corticosteroids (Addison's disease)

The patient may present as an emergency, with a low blood-pressure, dehydration, and pigmentation in the buccal mucosa. The electrolyte pattern is characteristic: the sodium concentration is low, the potassium concentration is high, and the urea level is high (due to the dehydration); the blood-sugar may be low.

To make a diagnosis it is recommended that while the patient is being hydrated with intravenous normal saline, a short synacthen test is carried out. A blood-sample is first taken for cortisol estimation. The patient is given 250 mg synacthen intravenously or intramuscularly and another blood-sample is taken 30 minutes after the synacthen injection for determination of the cortisol level. The cortisol level is low and does not respond to synacthen in a patient with Addison's disease. The patient can then be given hydrocortisone intravenously in order to raise the cortisol level; the diagnosis cannot be made after hydrocortisone is given.

Congenital adrenal hyperplasia

The commonest enzyme defect causing congenital adrenal hyperplasia is the 21-hydroxylase deficiency (see Chapter 4).

For the diagnosis of 11β- and the 21-hydroxylase deficiency infants should be more than 48 hours old. The plasma corticotrophin level is markedly raised. Plasma 17α-hydroxyprogesterone is also raised, and as there is normally a circadian variation in the plasma levels, a morning sample should be taken. In

Table 12.7 An example of hormone levels in congenital adrenal hyperplasia (21-hydroxylase deficiency): an adult female patient who presented with virilism

	Cortisol (nmol/l)	Testosterone (nmol/l)	17α-hydroxyprogesterone (nmol/l)
Basal blood sample a.m.	430 (NR 250–750)	19·9 (NR 0·5–2·5)	480 (NR up to 15)
250 mg synacthen given			
30 minutes post-synacthen	410	20·9	410
24-hour urine analysis			
17-oxosteroids	263 μmol (NR 15–70 μmol)		
Free cortisol	168 nmol (NR up to 275 nmol)		
Pregnanetriol	297 μmol (NR 1·5–7·5 μmol)		

NR = Normal range.

congenital adrenal hyperplasia the plasma 17α-hydroxyprogesterone level increases much more than in normal subjects after synacthen stimulation. The urinary level of pregnanetriol, a metabolite of 17α-hydroxyprogesterone, is also raised. The 11-oxygenation index (measured after at least 8 days of life) is increased above 0·5 in this condition.

Thyroid function

Suspected hyperthyroidism (thyrotoxicosis)

Measurement of total plasma T_4 and T_3 concentrations usually confirm the diagnosis. Estimations of the basal plasma thyrotrophin concentration are of no diagnostic value for thyrotoxicosis because it is not possible to measure low levels of this hormone. An example of values found in a patient with thyrotoxicosis is given in Table 12.8.

Table 12.8   Example of hormone levels in a patient with thyrotoxicosis

	Levels in patient	Normal range
Plasma T_4	180 nmol/l	60–160 nmol/l
Plasma T_3	12·5 nmol/l	1·4–3·0 nmol/l

In a mild or early thyrotoxicosis case it may be necessary to do a thyrotrophin releasing hormone (TRH) test.

TRH TEST: No preparation of the patient is required. It is preferable to do the test in the morning. A blood-sample is taken using a plain tube, and then 200 μg TRH is given as an intravenous bolus. Blood-samples are then taken 20 and 60 minutes after the injection. The 20-minute blood-sample should normally have a thyrotrophin level which has increased by at least 3 mU/l, to reach a value of 9 ± 3 (S.D.) mU/l. Table 12.9 is an example of the values for T_4, T_3, and thyrotrophin to be found in a patient with mild (or early) thyrotoxicosis.

Table 12.9   Example of hormone levels in mild (or early) thyrotoxicosis

	Levels in patient	Normal range
T_4 (nmol/l)	152	60–160
T_3 (nmol/l)	5·5	1·4–3·0
TRH test		
Thyrotrophin: basal (mU/l)	<2	up to 5
20-minute post TRH (mU/l)	<2	9 ± 3 (S.D.)
60-minute post TRH (mU/l)	<2	

Table 12.10 gives an example of the blood-levels in a female patient on the contraceptive pill or in pregnancy. In these circumstances the free T_3 and T_4 levels are normal, although total hormone levels (i.e. free hormone and

Table 12.10 Example of hormone levels in a female patient with raised total T_3 and T_4 levels due to the 'pill' or pregnancy

	Levels in patient	Normal range
T_4 (nmol/l)	170	60–160
T_3 (nmol/l)	3·9	1·4–3·0
TRH test:		
Thyrotrophin: basal (mU/l)	3	up to 5
20-minute post TRH (mU/l)	7	
60-minute post TRH (mU/l)	5	

hormone bound to thyroxine-binding globulin TBG) are raised. The TBG concentration may be measured directly and shown to be raised. The free thyroxine index which indirectly allows for the raised TBG level, will be normal. In patients with low TBG concentration (e.g. with nephrotic syndrome) the total T_3 and T_4 levels will be low but the free hormone concentrations will be normal. Thyrotrophin levels and the response to the TRH test will also be normal.

Suspected hypothyroidism (myxoedema)

Measurements of total T_4 and thyrotrophin levels are made. In most myxoedema patients the T_4 is less than 60 nmol/l and thyrotrophin is greater than 20 mU/l. The serum cholesterol level is raised. The TRH test would show an exaggerated response and does not add to the diagnosis. Table 12.11 gives an example of values found in myxoedema. One subgroup of patients has how-

Table 12.11 Example of hormone levels in a patient with myxoedema

	Levels in patient	Normal range
T_4 (nmol/l)	<10	60–160
Thyrotrophin (mU/l)	73	up to 5

Table 12.12 Two examples of hormone levels in pre-myxoedema

	Example 1	Example 2
T_4 (nmol/l)	85	113
T_3 (nmol/l)	2·5	1·9
TRH test		
Thyrotrophin: basal (mU/l)	10	5
20-minute post TRH (mU/l)	44	48
60-minute post TRH (mU/l)	37	39

ever been shown to have normal T_3 and T_4 levels but raised thyrotrophin levels, and this group of patients has been classified as premyxoedema, or subclinical hypothyroidism. These patients have a history of thyroid ablation and have positive thyroid antibodies. They show an exaggerated response to the TRH test, with or without a raised basal thyrotrophin level. Table 12.12 gives two examples of thyroid function test results in patients with premyxoedema. One patient had a high basal thyrotrophin level while the other had a normal basal level.

Hypothyroidism due to hypopituitarism

Thyroid function (together with adrenal cortex function) is one of the last functions to be affected in hypopituitarism. The T_4 and thyrotrophin levels are low, and there is usually no thyrotrophin response to the TRH test. Hypopituitarism is usually indicated by other evidence (see section on adenohypophysial function). Table 12.13 gives the hormonal levels found in a patient with hypopituitarism, showing hypothyroidism. In this example, the basal levels for T_4, T_3, thyrotrophin, testosterone, cortisol, LH, and FSH are all low. There is no response to TRH by thyrotrophin or prolactin.

Table 12.13 Example of hormone levels in a patient with hypopituitarism showing hypothyroidism

Time (min) after TRH test	T_4 (nmol/l)	T_3 (nmol/l)	TSH (mU/l)	PRL (mU/l)	Testosterone (nmol/l)	Cortisol (nmol/l)	LH (U/l)	FSH (U/l)
0	27	1·1	3	70	4·9	<25	<1·0	0·9
20			3	82				
60			3	70				

TSH = Thyrotrophin   PRL = Prolactin

Gonadal function

One cause of decreased gonadal function is hypopituitarism, which has been considered earlier in this chapter. It is useful to remember that gonadal function is the first to be affected by a developing pituitary tumour.

Decreased gonadal function in the female

Primary amenorrhoea

There are various causes of primary amenorrhoea (see Chapter 5). Blood levels found in one example, Turner's syndrome, are given in Table 12.14. In this example the patient was a girl of 16 with delayed puberty. The chromosome karyotype was XO. An LHRH test was carried out (as described previously) and the results are given in the Table.

Table 12.14 Example of hormone levels in a female patient (aged 16) with Turner's syndrome

Basal levels (0 time):
LH	27·2 U/l
FSH	49·5 U/l
oestrogen	57 pmol/l

LHRH test
20 minutes post LHRH test:
LH	>64 U/l
FSH	>50 U/l

Secondary amenorrhoea (infertility)

To investigate this condition a serum hormone profile is obtained. This consists of estimations of T_4, T_3, thyrotrophin, prolactin, oestradiol, progesterone, LH, and FSH concentrations. (Thyroid disease is excluded.)

CAUSES:

Post-pill amenorrhoea. Table 12.15 gives an example of the hormone profile in a female patient with 'post-pill' amenorrhoea. Secondary amenorrhoea is treated by Clomiphene (Chapter 5), and a blood-sample should be taken 21 days after the first dose of the drug. If ovulation has occurred the serum progesterone level will be above 10 nmol/l (luteal phase).

Table 12.15 Example of hormone levels in patient with 'post-pill' amenorrhoea

T_4	89 nmol/l
T_3	2·2 nmol/l
Thyrotrophin	3 mU/l
Prolactin	180 mU/l
Progesterone	<1·0 nmol/l†
Oestradiol	363 pmol/l
LH	14·5 U/l
FSH	6·7 U/l

† Normal progesterone range: follicular phase: up to 5 nmol/l; luteal phase: 10–60 nmol/l.

Polycystic ovary syndrome. Another cause of secondary amenorrhoea is polycystic ovary syndrome, and an example of the hormone profile in a patient with this condition is given in Table 12.16. The testosterone level is raised and the LH and FSH concentrations may be normal or high.

Possible pituitary tumour or 'microadenomata'. Secondary amenorrhoea may be caused by a pituitary tumour or microadenomata. Table 12.17 shows an example of the hormone profile of a female patient who had secondary amenorrhoea for 9 years but no galactorrhoea. In this patient no pituitary tumour was demonstrated using conventional radiography. As can be seen

Table 12.16   Example of hormone levels in a patient with polycystic ovary syndrome

T_4	73 nmol/l
T_3	1·3 nmol/l
Thyrotrophin	<2 mU/l
Prolactin	170 mU/l
Testosterone	15.3 nmol/l†
Oestradiol	368 pmol/l
Progesterone	<1·0 nmol/l
LH	28·6 U/l
FSH	5·8 U/l

† Normal female range 1·4–3·0 nmol/l.

from the Table, the prolactin level was very high while the LH and FSH concentrations were low. There was no LH or FSH response to LHRH. Treatment of this patient consisted of bromocriptine which resulted in restoration of prolactin levels to within the normal range, and the patient now appears to have started menstruating.

Table 12.17   Example of secondary amenorrhoea hormone levels in a patient with amenorrhoea classified as due to 'possible pituitary tumour or microadenomata'

T_4	66nmol/l
T_3	1·9 nmol/l
Thyrotrophin	2 mU/l
Prolactin	36 000 mU/l
Oestradiol	266 pmol/l
Testosterone	1·6 nmol/l
Progesterone	<1·0 nmol/l
LH	1·7 U/l
FSH	0·4 U/l

Premature ovarian failure. In patients with this condition the serum oestradiol concentration is low, while the LH, and especially the FSH, levels are high.

Decreased gonadal function in the male

CAUSES:

Hyperprolactinaemia. Some patients have raised serum prolactin levels and this should indicate a full investigation for a hypophysial (pituitary) tumour. Such patients respond to treatment with bromocriptine.

Some patients have testicular failure and on investigation are found to have low plasma testosterone but raised FSH and LH levels. Patients with hypopituitarism will have low testosterone, FSH, and LH plasma concentrations.

Klinefelter's syndrome. Patients with primary hypogonadism usually present with eunuchoidism and occasionally gynaecomastia. One cause of this condition is Klinefelter's syndrome, an example the hormone profile of which is shown in Table 12.18. In Klinefelter's syndrome patients, the degree of masculinization is dependent on the level of testosterone. An LHRH test is done on the patient first and confirmation is obtained by investigating the chromosome karyotype.

Table 12.18   Example of hormone levels in a male patient with Klinefelter's syndrome (karyotype XXY)

Basal plasma concentrations:
Testosterone   2·9 nmol/l†
     LH   24·5 U/l
    FSH   17·0 U/l

LHRH test
20 minutes post LHRH test:
     LH   62·7 U/l
    FSH   42.6 U/l
60 minutes post LHRH test:
     LH   57·4 U/l
    FSH   18·2 U/l

† Normal range 13–30 nmol/l.

Kallman's syndrome. Patients with this condition often have an associated anosmia and a family history of hypogonadism. The hypogonadism is due to isolated deficiency of LHRH. To investigate Kallman's syndrome, an LHRH test is carried out; an example of the hormone levels found with such a test in a patient with Kallman's syndrome is given in Table 12.19.

Points to note are that clomiphene has no effect on gonadotrophin release in these patients, and that treatment in the future will be LHRH therapy.

Table 12.19   Example of blood levels in a male patient with Kallman's syndrome

Basal hormone levels:
Testosterone   1·3 nmol/l
     LH   2·2 U/l
    FSH   0·7 U/l

LHRH test
20 minutes post LHRH test:
     LH   4·1 U/l
    FSH   1·5 U/l
60 minutes post LHRH test:
     LH   4·7 U/l
    FSH   2·0 U/l

Pancreatic function

Insulinoma

ESTIMATION OF BLOOD-GLUCOSE: The investigation of a patient with an insulinoma consists of taking a morning blood-sample after a 15-hour overnight fast, and repeating this procedure for two or three consecutive mornings. The blood-glucose concentration is measured in each sample and if it is below 2·2 mmol/l the serum insulin level is also measured. A serum insulin concentration greater than 10 mU/l in the presence of a hypoglycaemia is indicative of an insulinoma. Alternatively the patient can be fasted for 3 days and blood-glucose and insulin levels measured in samples taken each morning and evening. This more drastic procedure is seldom necessary since most patients with insulinomas develop hypoglycaemia within 24 hours.

Other tests include the glugacon test and the tolbutamide test.

GLUCAGON TEST: On the day of test, the patient should not be given food or water. Just before giving the glucagon, a blood-sample should be taken for blood-glucose and insulin estimations. The glucagon is then given intravenously through an indwelling catheter in a dose of 1 mg, and 10 ml blood-samples taken every 5 minutes for 20 minutes, then 30 minutes after administration and for the subsequent 30-minute period. One blood-sample is taken for each of the following 2 hours. The samples are then used for blood-glucose and serum insulin concentration measurements. If hypoglycaemic symptoms develop (e.g. sweating, vomiting, violence, semi-coma) a blood-sample is taken for the estimations of blood-glucose and insulin levels and the test is terminated. The patient is given 50 ml of 50% glucose intravenously and as soon as possible more glucose is given orally. As soon as the test is finished, the patient should be given food and water.

TOLBUTAMIDE TEST: This test may be used if the previous test has been inconclusive. On the day of test the patient should not be given food or water until after the test has been terminated. The procedure is similar to that described for the glucagon test. The dose of tolbutamide used is 1 g. Again it is necessary to take the precaution of having 50 ml of 50% glucose solution readily available for rapid intravenous administration should hypoglycaemic symptoms develop.

Diabetes mellitus

GLUCOSE TOLERANCE TEST: To diagnose this condition a glucose tolerance test (GTT) is used as described in the section on somatotrophin. The test is carried out in the morning, and an additional collection of urine 2 hours after the glucose administration, is made. In Table 12.20 examples of the changes in blood-glucose levels observed in a normal subject and a patient with diabetes mellitus are given. The normal ranges of blood-glucose concentrations given are the criteria of the British Diabetic Association. Some points to note from Table 12.20 are that no glucose was found in the 2-hour urine sample from the normal subject, whereas it was in the urine of the diabetic. The fasting blood-

Table 12.20   Examples of normal and diabetic blood-glucose levels (mmol/l) during the glucose tolerance test

	Diabetic patient	Normal subject	Normal range
Fasting	7·4	4·2	3–5
30 minutes after glucose	14·2	6·6	
60 minutes after glucose	14·9	8·0	below 8·9
90 minutes after glucose	15·1	6·8	
120 minutes after glucose	12·9	5·9	below 6·1

glucose level of the diabetic is high and the peak blood-glucose concentration is above the renal threshold. The 2-hour blood-glucose level has not dropped below 6·1 mmol/l.

The diabetic GTT response is usually due to insulin deficiency but may be caused by excess insulin-antagonizing hormones such as somatotrophin (see acromegaly), adrenalin (phaeochromocytoma), or cortisol (Cushing's syndrome).

The lag-response: Occasionally, a lag GTT response is observed, with results similar to those given in Table 12.21. In this type of response, the blood-glucose concentration rises rapidly above renal threshold to a peak and then falls equally rapidly. The lag GTT response may be seen in post-gastrectomy patients or in very severe liver disease, and rarely in thyrotoxicosis and in some normal individuals.

Table 12.21   Example of blood-glucose levels (mmol/l) showing a lag GTT response

Fasting blood glucose	4·1
30 minutes after glucose	9·4
60 minutes after glucose	9·6
90 minutes after glucose	6·7
120 minutes after glucose	3·9

The flat response: A flat GTT response may be seen in patients with malabsorption. However, it can also be found in normal subjects, and occasionally in patients with Addison's disease or hypopituitarism. Table 12.22 gives an example of a flat GTT response.

Table 12.22   An example of blood-levels (mmol/l) showing a flat GTT response

Fasting blood glucose	4·0
30 minutes after glucose	4.8
60 minutes after glucose	4·4
90 minutes after glucose	4·5
120 minutes after glucose	4·7

Parathyroid gland function

Hypoparathyroidism

This condition is relatively rare. Patients present with tetany and low serum calcium levels. On investigation, these patients have hypocalcaemia, hyper-phosphataemia, hypocalcuria, and occasionally hypophospaturia. Estimations of serum PTH levels may be of value but usually low levels, even in the normal range, cannot be detected.

Patients with idiopathic hypoparathyroidism show an increase in both urinary and plasma cyclic AMP levels after the administration of parathormone, while patients with pseudo-hypoparathyroidism show no such increases. High plasma concentrations of 25-hydroxycholecalciferol (25-OH vitamin D), such as values over 600 nmol/l (normal range 10–100 nmol/l) establish the diagnosis of vitamin D intoxication.

Hyperparathyroidism

Diagnosis of hyperparathyroidism is made on the basis of serum and urinary electrolyte levels, and on serum PTH levels. Chloride and calcium concentrations in the serum are raised while phosphate levels are reduced. In the urine calcium and phosphate excretion is increased. The PTH concentration is raised from a normal value of anything up to 0·73 μg/l to values as high as 1·2 μg/l.

Occasionally it is difficult to distinguish between the hypercalcaemia due to hyperparathyroidism from other causes such as carcinoma of the bronchus or breast. A useful differential test is the hydrocortisone test. Hydrocortisone does not usually suppress calcium levels in hyperparathyroidism (in 90 per cent of such patients) whereas it will lower calcium levels in some 60 per cent of patients suffering from the 'other causes'.

The test takes several days, so the patient must first adjust to the hospital ward environment. Once the patient has settled down, the test is begun. An initial blood-sample is taken and the patient is then given 40 mg of hydrocortisone every eight hours for at least 10 days. One blood-sample is taken each day between 0900 and 1000 hours with the patient fasting. From the twelfth or thirteenth day of test, the drug dose is gradually reduced until by the seventeenth day the drug therapy has ceased completely. In patients with hyperparathyroidism, the serum calcium level usually fluctuates around the mean (basal) value. In many of the patients with hypercalcaemia due to other causes, the serum calcium level will fall by 0·25–1 mmol/l.

REFERENCE TABLES

Normal levels of hormones in blood

Hormone		Value	Some useful conversions from SI units
Plasma aldosterone	Normal Na$^+$, K$^+$ diet (Na$^+$: 100–200 mmol/24 h; K$^+$: 50–80 mmol/24 h)	200–800 pmol/l	1 pmol/l ≈ 2·77 pg/ml
Plasma cortisol	0900 h	250–700 nmol/l	1 nmol/l ≈ 0.0362 μg/100 ml
	2400 h	up to 200 nmol/l	
Plasma corticotrophin (ACTH)	0800 h	40–120 ng/l	
	2000 h	< 5–50 ng/l	
Serum follicle stimulating hormone (FSH)	*Children* (1 year to puberty)	less than 2·5 U/l	
	Adult males	1–7 U/l	
	Adult females: Premenopausal Mid-cycle peak Postmenopausal	1–10 U/l 6–25 U/l 30–120 U/l	
Serum luteinizing hormone (LH)	*Male*	1·5–10 U/l	
	Female: Early follicular Mid-follicular Mid-cycle peak Luteal	2·5–15 U/l up to 20 U/l 5–70 U/l up to 13 U/l	
Serum 17β oestradiol	*Male*	Less than 200 pmol/l	1 pmol/l ≈ 0·27 pg/ml
	Female: Follicular Mid-follicular Luteal phase Postmenopausal	75–200 pmol/l 350–1500 pmol/l 200–1100 pmol/l less than 200 pmol/l	
Serum progesterone	Follicular	up to 5·0 nmol/l	1 nmol/l ≈ 0·32 ng/ml
	Luteal	10–60 nmol/l	
Plasma 17α-hydroxyprogesterone	Morning sample	up to 15 nmol/l	
Serum prolactin		up to 800 mU/l	
Plasma parathyroid hormone (PTH)		up to 0·73 μg/l	
Serum testosterone	*Male*	13–30 nmol/l	1 nmol/l ≈ 0·29 ng/ml
	Female	0·5–2·5 nmol/l	

Normal levels of hormones in blood *(continued)*

Hormone		Value	Some useful conversions from SI units
Plasma renin activity (PRA)	Normal Ha$^+$, K$^+$ diet (Na$^+$: 100–200 mmol/24 h; K$^+$: 50–80 mmol/24 h)	0·5–2·0 pmol/h/ml	
Serum thyrotrophin (TSH)		up to 5 mU/l	
Serum thyroxine (T$_4$)		60–160 nmol/l	1 nmol/l ≈ 0·8 ng/ml
Serum tri-iodothyromine (T$_3$)		1·4–3·0 nmol/l	1 nmol/l ≈ 0·6 ng/ml
Plasma 25-hydroxycholecalciferol (25-hydroxy vitamin D)		15–100 nmol/l	1 nmol/l ≈ 0·4 ng/ml
Plasma Vasopressin (AVP)		1–2 mU/l	1 mU/l ≈ 0·4 pg/ml

Normal levels of hormones excreted in urine in 24 hours

Hormone		Value	Some useful conversions from SI units
Aldosterone	Normal Na$^+$, K$^+$ diet (Na$^+$: 100–200 mmol/24 h; K$^+$: 50–80 mmol/24 h)	200–800 pmol/l	1 pmol/l ≈ 2·77 pg/ml
Free cortisol		up to 275 nmol	
Total oestrogens	*Male*	25–85 nmol	
	Female: Follicular Ovulatory peak Luteal	25–100 nmol 140–340 nmol 100–340 nmol	
17-oxogenic steroids	*Male*	15–70 μmol	1 μmol ≈ 0·29 mg
	Female	15–60 μmol	
17-oxosteroids	*Male*	15–85 μmol	1 μmol ≈ 0·29 mg
	Female	15–70 μmol	
Pregnanetriol	*Male*	3–6 μmol	1 μmol ≈ 0·33 mg
	Female	1·5–7·5 μmol	
Dehydropiandrosterone (DHA)	*Male*	0·35–7 μmol	
	Female	0·7–1·75 μmol	
Vanillyl mandelic-acid (VMA)		less than 40 μmol	

References

Selected background reading

Banting, F. G. and Best, C. H. (1922). The internal secretion of the pancreas. *J. Lab. clin. Med.* **7**, 251–66.

Harris, G. W. (1955). *Neural control of the pituitary gland*. Monographs of the physiological Society, No. 3. London.

Jacob, F. and Monod, J. (1961). Genetic regulatory mechanism in the synthesis of protein. *J. mol. Biol.* **3**, 318–56.

Starling, E. H. (1905). The Croonian lectures. *Lancet* **2**, 339–41; 423–5.

Verney, E. B. (1947). The antidiuretic hormone and the factors which determine its release. *Proc. Roy. Soc. B* **135**, 25–106.

Selected further reading

Hall, R., Anderson, J., Smart, G. A., and Besser, M. (1974). *Fundamentals of clinical endocrinology* (2nd edn). Pitman Medical, London.

Williams, R. H. (ed.) (1974). *Textbook of endocrinology* (5th edn). W. B. Saunders, Philadelphia.

Goodman, L. S. and Gilman, A. (1975) *The pharmacological basis of therapeutics* (5th edn). Macmillan, New York.

'Clinics in endocrinology and metabolism': series published annually by W. B. Saunders, Philadelphia.

Endocrine diseases. In *Medicine* (London) 2nd series 7–9 (1975 *et seq*.).

Guyton, A. C. and McCann, S. M. (1974). Endocrine physiology. *MIP International review of Science*, Series 1, vol. 5. Butterworths, London

Endocrinology. Section 7 of *Handbook of physiology*. The American Physiological Society (1972).

Selected recent reviews

Dousa, T. P. and Valtin, H. (1976). Cellular actions of vasopressin in the mammalian kidney. *Kidney International* **10**, 46–63.

Gerich, J. E., Charles, M. A., and Grodsky, G. M. (1976). Regulation of pancreatic insulin and glucagon secretion. *Ann. Rev. Physiol.* **38**, 353–88.

Sterling, K. and Lazarus, J. H. (1977). The thyroid and its control. *Ann. Rev. Physiol.* **39**, 349–72.

Vale, W., Rivier, C., and Brown, M. (1977). Regulatory peptides of the hypothalamus. *Ann. Rev. Physiol* **39**, 473–527.

Index